Testimonials for *Healthy You!*

"Thanks to *Healthy You!* I was able to reach a number on the scale that I haven't seen in years! I simply can't describe how GREAT I feel after being on the program for a full two weeks."

— Callie C, 30

"After reading *Healthy You!* I am more conscious of what and how I eat. I realize now how important it is to be attentive and make sure my diet is as balanced as my lifestyle. Since reading the book, I've lost 16 pounds and feel 10 years younger. This book changed my relationship with food and I'm never going back!"

—Mary H, 57

"After gaining 20 pounds over the last two years, I decided it was time to do something about it. Having never tried a weight loss program before, I was a bit skeptical; but after losing 10 pounds in just 5 days, I was sold!"

—Nathan C, 30

"I lost 6 pounds in the first week of the program! My appetite has dramatically reduced and my sugar and salt cravings are gone! The program is so easy to follow and has been simple to incorporate it into my schedule and lifestyle."

—Kelly B, 37

"In the past, I lost weight only to gain it back again and then some. It wasn't until I tried the *Healthy You!* program that I was able to shed the pounds and keep them off. During the 14 days, I lost over 12 pounds and have not only kept the weight off for months but have continued to lose even more weight by following the principles of the program."

ℳℴtt D, 46

"With the *Healthy You!* 　　　　　　　　tart my
weight loss! The progra𝗇 　　　　　　　　plateau
and I am now within 5 𝟙　　　　　　　　

.ia S, 38

Healthy You!

Healthy You!

*14 Days to Quick and Permanent Weight Loss
and a Healthier, Happier You*

Dawna Stone

HealthyYouVentures, LLC
P.O. Box 146
Saint Petersburg, FL 33731

Printed in the United States of America

First Edition: October 2013
10 9 8 7 6 5 4 3 2 1

ISBN 978-0615899664

Cover and interior design by Melissa Mellert

This publication is intended to provide helpful and informative material and is not intended to treat, diagnose, prevent or cure any health condition, nor is it intended to replace the advice of a physician. Always consult your physician before adopting a new eating or exercise regimen. The author and publisher specifically disclaim all responsibility for any liability, loss or risk, personal or otherwise, which is incurred as a consequence of reading or following advice or suggestions in this book.

Trademarked names are used throughout the book. Instead of placing a trademark symbol after every occurrence of a trademarked name, we use names in an editorial fashion only, with no intention of infringement of the trademark. Where such designations appear in the book, they have been printed with initial caps.

To Kaelie and Lucas

Table of Contents

Acknowledgments

Many people were instrumental in making this book a reality. First and foremost, I would like to thank my husband, Matt Dieter, for his patience, understanding and encouragement.

To my kids, Kaelie (6) and Lucas (4) who are still too young to truly understand the undertaking involved with writing a book. They have been a constant reminder of what's important in my life. I'll miss hearing them ask, "Mommy, are you still writing your book?"

I am extremely grateful to Ellen Madden, my friend and colleague at Healthy You Ventures and one of the hardest working individuals I know. I couldn't have finished the book without her support and encouragement.

Special thanks to my editor, Corinne Whiting. You were a pleasure to work with and the book is better because of you.

To Melissa Mellert, you are one of the most talented Art Directors I know. I was so fortunate to have you design the cover of the book.

I also want to thank the women who joined the Healthy You! focus group (Amelia, Amy, Ashley, Audrey, Callie, Cristin, Lauren, Mary, Michele, Molly and Stacey). Your feedback and suggestions were invaluable.

I want to thank my parents, my sister and my in-laws for believing in me.

Lastly, I thank you, my readers. May the HealthyYou! program help you lead the healthy and wonderful life you deserve.

Introduction

In 1985 the most commonly purchased women's dress size in America was an 8. Today it's climbed to a size 14, with nearly half of American women buying clothing in the plus-size category, often defined by retailers as sizes 14 to 34.

Everywhere you go, men and women seem to be uncomfortably bulging out of their clothing. But it's no longer just about how we look. Excess weight has become a health-eroding epidemic. The numbers astound. Obesity rates have more than doubled since the 1970s. Today more than two-thirds of Americans are overweight or obese.

As Americans continue to dine out more frequently, ingest more sugar and processed foods and prepare increased portion sizes, it's no wonder so many men and women are overweight and unhealthy.

Ironically, people today are more aware than ever of what they put into their bodies and how different foods can affect one's mood and health. But this increased knowledge only brings about positive change if people are willing to take action.

The Healthy You! program helps you ditch unhealthy habits, while building a foundation for well-balanced, wholesome eating that will not only facilitate your weight loss, but also lead to a longer, happier life.

By following the 14-day Healthy You! program, you can lose unwanted pounds and take the first step to a more vibrant and pleasurable existence. You can transform from someone whose body prevents them from living their best life to someone whose body propels them to new levels of happiness and well-being.

The Healthy You! program offers a plan for life. Although you can experience immediate weight loss on the plan, it's not a quick-fix fad diet maintainable only for a short period of time. Instead, it provides a whole new way of looking at food and health. The program gives you a simple-to-follow road map, allowing you to lose weight without depriving yourself of the foods you love. The easy-to-follow strategy promises immediate results that will keep you motivated while you achieve your long-term weight loss goals. As with any change in your diet or exercise routine, you should always consult a doctor before you begin.

I am confident that the Healthy You! program will work for you. Please share your success stories at dawnastone.com. The Healthy You! program changed my life, and I know it can change yours too!

PART ONE

Before You Begin

CHAPTER 1

Helpless to Hopeful

Years ago, I felt alone—like I was the only person who couldn't regulate my weight. My life was consumed by thoughts of food—the carton of ice cream in the freezer or the box of cookies in the cupboard. I didn't have control over my eating; food had taken control of me. If I knew then what I know now, I wouldn't have felt so helpless. I've since learned that millions of men and women confront similar issues on a daily basis. Over time, I found that by making a few simple changes, I could regain control of my eating, lose weight, get healthy and lead the life I'd always desired.

I didn't always know how to manage my weight or how to embrace healthier habits. Like so many, I spent years trying every diet in the book: no carb, no fat, juice fasting (I didn't make it past the first day), Scarsdale, the Grapefruit Diet, Jenny Craig and more only to find myself disappointed, irritable, depressed and often weighing more than when I had begun. I knew something had to change. Through trial and error, I eventually found the secret to controlling my eating and maintaining a healthy weight. That knowledge, which I'll share with you in the following chapters, forever changed my life. I only wish someone had shared the Healthy You! program with me long ago.

My battle with food really heated up in 1990, after I graduated from college and moved to New York City to work as a financial analyst for a Wall Street investment bank. Although I gained the typical "freshman 15" during my college years, I was still in reasonably decent shape when I moved to the Big Apple. But after graduation, it wasn't long before I stopped exercising completely and gained an additional 25 pounds.

The long hours demanded of my job, the late night pizza runs, the company cafeteria and the constant barrage of baked goods in the office (not to mention solo midnight trips to the corner market for my favorite indulgences) had me quickly outgrowing my clothes and feeling increasingly moody and tired. For the first time in my life, I was truly overweight.

I tried every "quick fix" to shed the pounds from jumping on the latest bandwagon diets and joining Jenny Craig to seeking help from a special weight loss clinic. Yet all these diets proved only temporarily effective. In the end, I gained a few additional pounds with each failed attempt. I was caught in a downward spiral, and I felt defeated.

I had all but given up on ever losing weight and feeling healthy again. Each failed diet left me lying tearfully in bed, convinced that my overweight body would never change. I no longer believed in my own ability to ever successfully lose weight or reach my ideal clothing size.

Did You Know?
You are not alone! According to the International Food Information Council Foundation's 2012 Food & Health Survey, more than half of all Americans are trying to lose weight.

Then one day, it dawned on me: the reason I couldn't lose weight—or keep off the weight I did lose—stemmed from using programs that weren't right for me. I didn't want to be weighed publicly in front of other people, and I didn't enjoy eating tiny, prepackaged meals. But I also didn't have time to fix the elaborate meals touted by some books and magazines. The eating plan designed for me by a bodybuilder (yes, I told you, I've tried it all!) worked for a short while, but I knew that, realistically, eating only chicken, tuna and vegetables wasn't a sustainable lifestyle I could enjoy. I needed variety in the foods I ate. Like most people, I truly enjoy eating, and I relish good food.

I finally had an epiphany: in order to find a weight loss program that offers me everything I want—the option to easily dine out, follow simple recipes, enjoy a variety of meals, occasionally indulge in my favorite foods and, most importantly, sustain the weight loss—I would need to develop my own system.

It took me many years to come up with an effective program that not only guarantees long-lasting results, but is also enjoyable to follow. The Healthy You! program is a culmination of years of research as well as years of testing countless other methods. Once I finally discovered a formula that worked, the weight started falling off and, more importantly, staying off. The results were quick and easy, and people in my life began to take notice. Some of my co-workers soon asked if I could help them with their own weight loss struggles. At the time, I had never thought of "my" program as something I would share with others. I simply developed it because I had grown fed up with following others' plans. But I soon realized that so many like myself had unsuccessfully attempted innumerable weight loss programs, and they too were frustrated.

I started sharing my program with co-workers, friends and family. I was willing to help anyone who asked. Once these initial participants began to lose weight, they introduced me to others who also sought my help. Soon I was sharing my healthy eating tips with local women's groups and clubs.

Although I was able to help an ever-expanding group of people, my career limited my ability to spread the word beyond a certain point. It wasn't until I left my corporate job and launched a sports and fitness magazine—initially called *Her Sports + Fitness* magazine and later rebranded *Women's Run-*

ning magazine—that I was able to share my ideas about weight loss, nutrition and physical activity with thousands of people. I wrote an inspirational Founder's Letter in each issue of the magazine. Thanks to the recognition I received with the magazine, I was then asked to do a segment on Fox News called "Healthy Living with Dawna Stone." I could finally share my healthful living tips with even more people. Although thousands of viewers and readers now heard my message, it wasn't enough. I still dreamt of further expanding my reach to help people everywhere.

A couple years later, a friend called and convinced me to try out for the TV reality series "The Apprentice: Martha Stewart." I never imagined being selected as a contestant, but to make a very long story short, I not only became one of the program's 16 candidates, but I also won the entire show and spent most of 2006 in New York City working with Martha. During that year, I was fortunate to have many new and exciting experiences, including landing my own weekly radio show on Sirius Satellite Radio called "Health and Fitness Talk with Dawna Stone." I also spent the year writing a regular healthy living column in *Body+Soul* magazine (now *Whole Living* magazine). I appeared as a frequent guest on the "MARTHA" television talk show, preparing healthy recipes from *Body+Soul* magazine on set and providing the audience with health-conscious tips. I even led a series of shows that focused on a weight loss makeover—by far some of my favorite segments to work on.

My collaboration with Martha provided an even bigger platform from which to spread my healthy living message. As my apprenticeship with Martha came to an end, I returned to my expanding media business. *Women's Running* magazine continued to grow, and I launched a national women's running series. Focusing on my two businesses didn't allow me to share my message as frequently as I would have liked, and I always imagined that I would someday find a way to once again help men and women lose weight and lead healthier lives.

In May of 2012, I sold both companies—*Women's Running* magazine and the Women's Half Marathon series, which had expanded to five running events across the country. The sale gave me the opportunity to pursue the next phase of my life. Today, through this book, I can share my HealthyYou! program with even more men and women!

My goal is to help you understand how you can once and for all control your eating, maintain a healthy weight and forever change your life for the better. HealthyYou! provides more than just a set of rules or tips; it's an easy to-follow program that will help you maintain your ideal body weight, while elevating many aspects of your life to whole new levels.

CHAPTER 2

The Benefits of the Healthy You! Program

While the primary goal of Healthy You! is to help you reach a healthy weight, it's also about leading an overall better life. I've spent the last 15 years—through my TV segments "Healthy Living with Dawna Stone," my Sirius radio show "Health and Fitness Talk with Dawna Stone," my numerous motivational talks and countless magazine articles—encouraging and inspiring people to lose weight and get healthy.

If you experience any or all of these symptoms:
- Lack energy or tire easily
- Suffer from frequent headaches
- Have trouble falling asleep or sleeping through the night
- Feel anxious or stressed
- Overeat or crave sugary or starchy foods
- Lack self-esteem
- Have digestive issues or chronic stomach pain
- Have dull or lackluster skin

the Healthy You! program is for you.

The Healthy You! program can not only help you lose weight but it can also help you:
- Increase your energy levels
- Sleep better
- Reduce stress and anxiety

- Manage cravings and mood swings
- Elevate self-esteem
- Improve digestion
- Enhance your complexion

Followed properly, the HealthyYou! program can be key in attaining optimal health.

HealthyYou! can be successfully employed in a great variety of situations. Whether you're trying to lose 10 to 20 pounds or are the constant dieter struggling to lose 50, 75 or 100+ pounds, you can utilize HealthyYou! as an ongoing resource for leading a healthier life and achieving permanent weight loss.

Did You Know?
The Centers for Disease Control and Prevention states that being overweight or obese may raise the risk of illness from high blood pressure, high cholesterol, heart disease, stroke, diabetes, certain types of cancer, arthritis and breathing problems.

The following chapters will help you develop the mindset necessary to obtain long-term success. Believing in yourself, staying positive and eliminating negative self-talk will not only aid in your weight loss, but can drastically improve all aspects of your life. Throughout the book, you'll find real-life anecdotes and actionable tips that will help you stay motivated and positive.

As you get ready to embark on the HealthyYou! program, you will also receive tips on how to remove foods that trigger you to overeat and how to find the support you need for success.

The Healthy You! 14-day program serves as the cornerstone of the book. This section discusses how the way you choose to fuel your body determines not only your weight, but also how you feel and act. It outlines what's wrong with the typical American diet and how clean eating can be the key to successful weight loss.

You will read about individuals who progressed from varying levels of unhealthiness to transforming their bodies; in the process, they learned to lead happier, healthier, more fulfilled lives. These men and women are not unlike you; they simply made the decision to take the first step toward better eating.

The Healthy You! weight loss program is divided into two one-week phases—the Elimination Phase and the Clean Phase. Each phase includes a detailed and easy-to-follow meal plan and accompanying recipes. These two weeks have been designed to help you reevaluate your food choices and to pave the way to a cleaner, healthier diet.

Once you complete the initial two-week plan, you can choose to continue with the Clean Phase regimen to drop even more weight, or you can take what you've learned and maintain a diet that's less restrictive, but still relatively clean.

You'll also find advice for implementing the Healthy You! program in the midst of real-world situations like dining out, attending holiday parties and balancing busy schedules. Any time your focus lies in making changes, the possibility arises of encountering roadblocks. This section of the book will help you overcome the potential challenges you'll experience along the way.

In addition to the regular 14-day Healthy You! program, you will have the option of choosing the accelerated program which can be found in Appendix II. Although this program also lasts for 14 days, it is slightly more intense and provides even quicker results.

While writing the book, I once again tested some of my own concepts, mixing in different variables. I wanted to see what would happen if I stayed on the Clean Phase for longer than one week, and I wanted to see what would happen if I followed the program without incorporating any exercise at all. I already knew firsthand that the two-week Healthy You!

program worked; after all, it had enabled me to finally achieve my goal weight after years of struggling with yo-yo dieting. It's also what had helped me to lose the 40 pounds I gained during my first pregnancy—and what allowed me to once again reach my goal weight after my second pregnancy. While writing this book, I found that the program gave such great results that I felt motivated to stay on the Clean Phase for longer than a week, leading to even more weight loss. More importantly, the program encouraged me to fully examine my eating habits and to make cleaner choices going forward.

I still believe that the most effective methods are the regular two-week Healthy You! program or the accelerated two-week Healthy You! program, as outlined in this book. However, I do believe that there is also such a thing as being too thin, and every reader must determine a healthy weight for her or his body. If you find yourself dropping too much weight on the program, you can always increase your serving sizes or include additional snacks or calories throughout the day.

While the initial program incorporates healthy meals and snacks, it also explains how to enjoy occasional indulgences after week two without sabotaging your weight loss goals. Going out to dinner and indulging in a decadent dessert without any guilt is an amazing feeling—one I never would have experienced without the Healthy You! program.

The Healthy You! program shows you how to finally obtain that incredible, lean and healthy body you've always dreamed of, without depriving yourself of the foods you love. It's the only program that worked for me, and I am confident it will work for you, too.

CHAPTER 3

Be Positive and Believe in Yourself!

Henry Ford said, "Whether you think you can or think you can't, you're right." There was a time when I didn't believe I could lose weight. I now know that not believing in myself proved almost as detrimental to my weight loss as not eating correctly. It wasn't until I began to truly envision myself losing the weight that I had the right mindset to set me on the path to success.

Even if you've tried every diet out there to no avail, you have to believe that it's possible to achieve the lean and healthy body you deserve. Let me give you an example.

I met Jennifer in 2006 during a makeover series I hosted on Martha Stewart's "MARTHA" television show. We were looking to feature a woman who had struggled with her weight and had all but given up. Jennifer was a mother of two who was fed up with being overweight, exhausted and unable to keep up with her daughters.

Before starting Jennifer on a new eating and exercise plan, we sent her to the doctor for a full physical. Although Jennifer knew she was somewhat overweight, she was shocked to learn that she was actually obese and that her weight left her at risk for heart disease, diabetes and multiple types of cancer. Jennifer was only 35 years old.

After following a new eating regimen that consisted of healthy meals and snacks, in addition to starting a simple exercise program, Jennifer lost nearly 40 pounds, experienced higher energy levels and felt proud of her new body. Not only had she successfully shed the unwanted weight, but she was now in the best shape of her life and able to keep pace with her daughters. As an added bonus, her husband lost nearly 20 pounds because of the family's newfound focus on making better meal choices.

In his international bestseller "The Power of Positive Thinking," Norman Vincent Peale writes: "Believe in yourself! Have faith in your abilities! Without a humble but reasonable confidence in your own powers, you cannot be successful or happy. But sound self-confidence leads to self-realization and successful achievement." Jennifer experienced a huge transformation, but the changes she made to her diet and activity level were minimal. It was the combined effect of several minor changes, along with the belief that she could finally lose weight that ultimately made the difference.

Ask Dawna

I've failed at so many diets that I just can't believe that anything will work for me. How can I even think about success, when all I've experienced is failure?

I get most excited when I get to help someone who has given up. I know what it's like to feel defeated, to not fit into your "fat" jeans and to look in the mirror and cry. But I also now know what it feels like to be thin and healthy, to enjoy eating dessert and to not worry about gaining weight. Don't give up on yourself. Make a commitment to this program, and believe that it can work for you. This can be "your" successful program and not just another failed attempt. Follow the program exactly as it's outlined. Followed correctly, I know you can lose weight.

After my speaking engagements, women often approach me seeking advice on how to feel healthier and look better. They want to feel the exuberance of youth again; they want to experience the same passion for life they once had. For many women, negative moods, job-related issues and relationship problems stem from how they feel about their bodies and overall well-being. These women confide in me about their lack of control around food, their negative body images and their countless failed attempts at dieting.

My heart breaks when I meet these women and hear their common plights. I sense that the excess weight they carry relates to much more than their bodies; they're imprisoned by emotional baggage. I sometimes find myself crying with these women—not only because I feel for them, but also because I know how they feel. I know how badly these women want to change, but first they must believe it's possible. They have to begin by treating themselves with more respect. Men often don't share their feelings about weight as openly as women, but this doesn't mean that they don't struggle as well. I know firsthand that it's difficult to feel good about yourself when you're not satisfied with your weight, but I also know that it's easier to change your eating habits once you believe in your own worth.

Ask Dawna
I have no willpower; how am I ever going to lose weight?

It's not willpower that is sabotaging your weight loss; it's negativity. It's impossible to lose weight if you don't believe you can do it. The first step to getting the body you want is having confidence that you can succeed. Stop thinking about willpower, and instead focus on the little changes you can make starting today.

Can you commit to drinking more water this week? How about eating a few more fruits and vegetables? How about a 15-minute walk or a 10-minute run? You probably have a lot more willpower than you give yourself credit for. Write down two or three minor changes that you can make this week that will get you headed down a healthier path. These baby steps will ultimately have you racing toward success!

Sadly, we are often the ones who sabotage our own weight loss without even realizing it. If you ask most people (particularly women) what they are most dissatisfied with, again and again you'll hear references to bodies and weight. From an early age, many of us are fixated on body image.

The first time I remember truly worrying about my weight, I was 12 years old. My swim coach made everyone on the team fill out a food log and review it with him at the end of each week. If just one of us didn't follow his strict eating guidelines, the entire team would be punished. During our punishment period, the coach continually reminded the team which person had been at fault.

Even worse than the extra workouts, the coach inflicted punishment on team members who he thought had gained weight. He considered being overweight a sign of weakness, and if he suspected you were guilty of this, he would demand that you run laps around the pool deck in your swimsuit, while the rest of the team watched from the bleachers. I wasn't overweight at the time, but I must have watched my friend Carolyn run hundreds of laps around the pool—the rest of us, boys included, looking on. I was terrified of gaining weight.

Looking back, no 12-year-old should be fixated on her weight. Yet today, many young girls and boys begin thinking about this at an even earlier age. A few years ago on my radio show "Health and Fitness Talk with Dawna Stone," I hosted a segment focusing on body image and self-esteem in young adults. A mother called in to discuss her daughter's obsession with being fat. The most alarming thing about the call? The daughter was only six years old and, according to her doctor, an appropriate weight for her age and height. Why was this young girl already concerned about being "too fat"?

In today's world, it's difficult to escape the media's portrayal of the "perfect woman"—someone who can do it all and have it all, while wearing a size two dress—and the "perfect man"—who features a chiseled body with six-pack abs. The expectations we face amid a thin-at-all-costs culture can be overwhelming and immobilizing, leaving many of us with dangerously negative self-perceptions.

No doubt, our weight and overall appearance directly affect how we feel about ourselves and the way we live our lives. As we age, our bodies change. We often become less active, lose muscle mass, gain weight and accumulate responsibilities like work, children and spouses that threaten to take precedence over our own self-care. Sometimes before we know it, we wake up one morning to find a body in the mirror that we no longer recognize.

The bigger problem: a negative self-image bleeds into many other aspects of life, stopping us from reaching our potential in areas from personal relationships to professional lives and, of course, also hindering weight loss goals. You may suddenly find you don't feel as sexy as you once did, you may get out of breath climbing a flight of stairs, or you might lack the energy to go that extra mile at work.

Did You Know?

According to Harvard researcher and positive psychology expert Shawn Achor, the positive brain is 31% more productive than when the brain is negative, neutral or stressed.

As you start the Healthy You! program, prepare to change the way you feel about yourself. Be kinder to yourself, stay positive, and believe that you're capable of reaching your weight loss goals. You can do anything you set your mind to!

Like Norman Vincent Peale, I believe that we are all capable of more than we can possibly imagine. If we expect great things, great things will happen.

As you embark on the Healthy You! program:
- Believe you can do it
- Remember that even small changes lead to big results
- Imagine yourself succeeding
- Leave past failures behind and start fresh today
- Make a commitment to the program and to your health
- Know that you're not alone

CHAPTER 4

Set Realistic Goals

Not surprisingly, weight loss always tops New Year's resolution lists. But merely setting the goal may not be enough. Before you embark on your weight loss journey, you need to clarify goal specifics.

Clearly Define Your Goal

Your weight loss goal needs to be well-defined and given an assigned time frame. For example, having a generic weight loss aim isn't as effective as articulating the goal to lose 45 pounds by March 1. The probability of achieving success increases when you hone in on a well-defined goal with a target end date. Making goals clear and specific helps you to achieve them.

Ask Dawna
I have a lot of weight to lose. Should I set short-term or long-term weight loss goals?

The answer is simple: BOTH. Any long-term goals should consist of milestones or a series of short-term goals. For example, your long-term goal may be to lose 40 pounds, but you should divide that end goal into smaller steps like losing 10 pounds by a certain date, 20 pounds by a later date, etc. Setting short-term goals makes your long-term goal easier to achieve.

Make it Realistic

Make sure you set realistic intentions. Your goal should be challenging but also achievable. There's nothing worse than setting yourself up for failure. Your goal should be one that gets you to a healthy weight for your body, disregarding futile hopes of resembling a supermodel or Hollywood superhero.

Write it Down and Make it Your Own

Write down your goal and refer back often. Mount it somewhere you'll see it on a regular basis. It might go without saying, but make sure that "your" goal is not someone else's. Too many people get sidetracked by what others want for (or of) them. You have to really want the goal. If your husband wants you to lose weight but you feel perfectly content as you are, the likelihood of achieving the goal is much lower than if you want the change for yourself.

Break it Down

If you have 30 or more pounds to lose, break down your total plan into stages. Each milestone or short-term goal will get you closer to your final mark, yet the process will feel less daunting. For example, attempt to lose the first 10 pounds by a certain date, the next 10 pounds by a later date and so on.

Review It

Review your goals on a regular basis and monitor your progress. Praise yourself when you're on track. If you happen to fall off, figure out what steps need to be taken to get moving in the right direction once again.

Share It

Share your goals with others. Just telling someone else about your ambitions makes them seem more real and makes you feel more accountable. It may also help you garner support for your goals, which will make the challenging days feel easier.

Adjust It

Weight loss doesn't always unfold exactly as we expect. For example, some people will lose a great deal of weight in the first few days of the program, while others may not see a huge drop in the scale until week two. Be prepared to reevaluate your goals, and make minor adjustments as needed along the way. Try not to get caught up comparing yourself to others.

Know Why It's Important

Write down why it's important for you to reach your goal. Maybe you simply want to eat healthier, maybe you want to have more energy to run around with your kids, or maybe you want to fit into your favorite pair of jeans. No matter the reasons for wanting to lose weight, exploring the root of the issue and seeing the answers in black and white will help keep you motivated.

Reward Yourself

Reward yourself for a job well done. If you have a goal of losing 50 pounds total, and you lose 10 within the first two weeks, celebrate yourself. Just make sure your reward is in line with your long-term weight loss goals (food may not be the best "prize," for example). Instead, reward yourself with a new pair of shoes or a smaller size pair of jeans, get your nails done, or buy yourself a new lipstick. It doesn't matter how big or small the reward, just acknowledge your hard work and the achievement.

Follow these 10 steps to help achieve your goal:
- Clearly define your goal
- Make it realistic
- Write it down
- Make sure it's "your" goal
- Break it down into smaller steps
- Review it on a regular basis

- Share it with others
- Make adjustments if needed
- Know why you want it
- Reward yourself

CHAPTER 5

Accept Setbacks and Move Forward

If you follow the day-by-day HealthyYou! meal plan, you will most likely see quick and constant weight loss during the 14-day program. If you have a substantial amount of weight to lose that will take longer than two weeks, don't let small setbacks derail your ultimate goal. It is normal for people to have ups and downs when trying to drop large amounts of weight. By anticipating some bumps along the way, you'll be better equipped to achieve a healthy weight without letting small discouragements permanently sideline you.

Most people think they should witness steady weight loss from day one. In their mind's eye, their weight loss should look like the chart below.

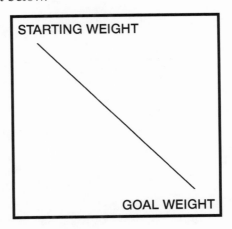

You may experience this type of weight loss during the 14-day Healthy You! program, but beyond the two weeks, your weight loss will probably fluctuate. Even with solid determination and hard work, someone can go from losing a few pounds at a steady pace to leveling out at a plateau for a short period. If you push forward, you can continue losing again after your body resets itself to the lower weight. You will still reach your end goal weight, but you'll likely enter a few phases where you're not losing weight, and you may even fluctuate by a few pounds. When this happens, just be patient and realize it's part of the process. Know that if you stick with the program, your body will once again respond to the positive changes you're making. A more realistic weight loss chart looks like this:

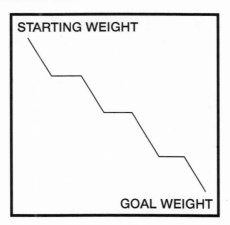

This reflects an initial stage of weight loss, followed by a plateau, followed by more weight loss and more plateaus, until you eventually achieve your goal weight.

The problem begins when people allow plateaus or temporary weight gains to throw them into emotional turmoil and they view the process as "all or nothing." This is what causes so many people to lose weight, only to gain it back within a relatively short period; an inability to flawlessly reach a goal weight is seen as a complete failure. Unfortunately when this happens, most people gain weight rather than lose as the chart depicts below.

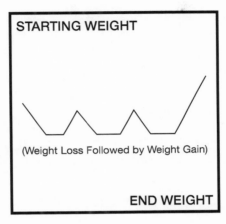

STARTING WEIGHT

(Weight Loss Followed by Weight Gain)

END WEIGHT

The chart below represents a realistic snapshot for individuals who have more than a few pounds to lose. By anticipating bumps in the road, you'll realize you can and will push past the plateau periods. Expect your weight loss chart to look something like this:

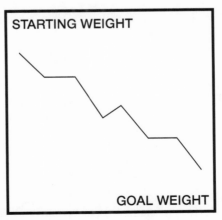

STARTING WEIGHT

GOAL WEIGHT

Factors like business travel, family vacations, stress or innocent "slip-ups" might temporarily derail you, but, regardless, it is important to not view your weight loss as an "all or nothing" pursuit.

CHAPTER 6

Who Are You?

Each of us is unique, and knowing who we truly are—our patterns, habits and quirks—can make sticking to a healthy eating program easier. Knowing your personality "profile" can prove as important as knowing your target goal weight. To get the most out of the program, you should follow the plan for your specific profile. Take a minute to read the following five descriptions, and determine which category best matches your personality. Are you a Remote Controller, Non-Believer, Flip Flopper, Food Abuser or Almost Achiever? Most of us will fall somewhere in between two groups, but one profile should be a closer fit than the rest. Find the one that best describes you, and read the five corresponding tips for your profile that will help ensure your success on the program.

During the many years I struggled with my weight and before following the Healthy You! program I developed, I would have best fit the profile of the Food Abuser. Because of my profile, the accelerated plan worked best for me and not only allowed me to lose weight quickly, but also helped me keep it off. Identify the appropriate profile for you, and follow the accompanying tips for your specific personality type.

The Remote Controller
The Remote Controller does a lot of unconscious eating. These people eat while watching TV, driving or working on the com-

puter, never realizing just how many extra calories they're ingesting. Weight gain happens at a steady pace, and the mindless eating becomes second nature.

The Remote Controller views exercise as too hard. It's just not for them. They can't fathom going to the gym or even finding 15 minutes during which to be active. The Remote Controller doesn't like to sweat nor does he or she want to put on exercise clothes. They only make the movements required for daily life, but even that is done without much energy. They know they need to change, but they don't know how to start, and they lack the motivation to learn. The remote controller often needs to lose 40 to 100 pounds (or more).

5 Tips for the Remote Controller:
1. Follow the regular 14-day Healthy You! program but stay on the clean phase (with occasional indulgences) until you reach your goal weight.
2. Eat only at the table.
3. Do not eat while doing other activities like watching TV, talking on the phone, driving, working, etc.
4. Keep a food log or journal.
5. Although not mandatory on the program, an exercise program would help accelerate the Remote Controller's weight loss. If you're not exercising already, take a 20 – 30 minute walk three or four times a week. If you're already exercising, add 15 more minutes to your current routine.

The Non-Believer

The Non-Believer threw out their "skinny jeans" years ago. There might have been a time that they believed they could lose weight, but those days are long gone. They don't exercise, yet they lead a moderately active lifestyle. Their lack of formal exercise and poor nutrition habits have led them to weight gain. The Non-Believer often needs to lose 30 – 60 pounds but can't imagine it ever happening for them. They've tried dieting without success and are fed up; they are resigned to being eternally overweight.

5 Tips for the Non-Believer:
1. For faster results, start with the accelerated plan.
2. Believe in yourself; stop the negative self-talk.
3. Keep a journal, and track your meals along with your progress.
4. Weigh yourself before you begin the program, and then wait until the end of week one to check your progress.
5. Begin a walking program, or incorporate moderate aerobic activity at least three days a week.

The Flip Flopper

The Flip Flopper lives on a roller coaster ride. They lose weight only for short periods and then gain it back again. They start an exercise program, aiming to finally stick to it, only to have their motivation peter out. They have great intentions, but very little follow-through. They keep "fat pants" and "skinny jeans" in their closet, but never seem to make it into their "skinny jeans" for long. The flip flopper does some exercise but never maintains a regular program. They lead a moderately active lifestyle but don't get enough exercise or stick to a healthy eating plan long enough to lose unwanted pounds. The Flip Flopper typically needs to lose 20 – 40 pounds.

5 Tips for the Flip Flopper:
1. Follow the regular 14-day Healthy You! program.
2. Keep track of your meals and your progress in a journal.
3. Enlist a friend, family member or colleague to do the program with you.
4. Partake in physical activity five days a week for a minimum of 30 minutes. If financially feasible, hire a trainer, or exercise with a friend at a set time each day.
5. Weigh yourself before you begin the program, and then

wait until the end of week one to check your progress.

The Food Abuser

The Food Abuser could easily achieve their goals if only they took control of their diet. Typically poor nutrition habits rather than a lack of exercise keep the extra weight around. The Food Abuser is moderately active but carries extra weight and often needs to lose 20 – 40 pounds. Their active lifestyle is the only thing preventing them from gaining additional weight.

5 Tips for the Food Abuser:
1. For faster results, start with the accelerated plan.
2. Remove all junk food from your house for the duration of the program.
3. Drink plenty of water throughout the day to curb junk food cravings.
4. Keep track of your meals and progress in a journal.
5. Keep snacks to one per day. It may be helpful to move the snack scheduled between lunch and dinner to post-dinner.

The Almost Achiever

The Almost Achiever's goal is within reach, but they just can't seem to do what it takes to get there. No matter how hard they try, they can't manage to lose those last few pounds. They typically want to lose only 5 – 15 pounds. The Almost Achiever not only leads an active lifestyle, but he or she also exercises regularly. Small changes in their eating habits will help them finally achieve their goal and their perfect weight.

5 Tips for the Almost Achiever:
1. Follow the regular 14-day Healthy You! program.
2. Track your meals and progress in a journal.
3. If you don't already have one, find an exercise partner, and increase current exercise program by 15 minutes per workout.

4. Focus on portion control; since you only need to lose 5 to 10 pounds, simply cutting back on serving sizes can help you achieve your goal in record time.
5. Weigh yourself on a daily basis for the entire two-week period.

Once you know your personality type, use that knowledge along with the tips provided to help you on your path to weight loss success.

PART TWO

The Healthy You! Program

CHAPTER 7

The Elimination Phase

As you've learned by now, the HealthyYou! program has allowed me to maintain a healthy body and an ideal weight for over ten years. The simple-to-follow plan with its immediate results will keep you motivated during the entire 14 days.

The HealthyYou! weight loss program consists of two one-week phases—the Elimination Phase and the Clean Phase. Each phase includes a detailed and easy-to-follow meal plan and accompanying recipes. These two weeks have been designed to help you reevaluate your food choices and to get you started on a cleaner, healthier diet.

Once you complete the two weeks, you can choose to continue on the Clean Phase and drop even more weight, or you can take what you've learned and eat a less restrictive diet that's still relatively clean.

During the Elimination Phase, participants focus on restricting one new item or category from his or her diet each day. At the end of the seven days, all seven items should have been completely eliminated from the diet. During this week, you will gradually drop sugar, wheat, dairy, highly processed foods, diet sodas and artificial sweeteners, red meat and alcohol. Don't worry, remember that the HealthyYou! program doesn't restrict any foods for the long-term.

Eliminating these foods will, however, allow you to focus on those healthy foods often overlooked in our diets like fresh fruits and vegetables, healthy grains and beans. It will also help you better understand how these eliminated foods have been making you feel. At the end of the seven days, your diet will consist of nothing but healthy, clean foods. Use the chart below as your guide during the Elimination Phase.

Week 1: The Elimination Phase (Days 1 – 7)

Day 1: Eliminate Sugar

Day 2: Eliminate Wheat (Plus Sugar)

Day 3: Eliminate Dairy (Plus Sugar and Wheat)

Day 4: Eliminate Highly Processed Foods (Plus Sugar, Wheat and Dairy)

Day 5: Eliminate Diet Soda and Artificial Sweeteners (Plus Sugar, Wheat, Dairy and Highly Processed Foods)

Day 6: Eliminate Red Meat (Plus Sugar, Wheat, Dairy, Highly Processed Foods and Diet Soda and Artificial Sweeteners)

Day 7: Eliminate Alcohol (Plus Sugar, Wheat, Dairy, Highly Processed Foods, Diet Soda and Artificial Sweeteners and Red Meat)

Follow the plan as closely as possible. On day one eliminate all unnatural sugar from your diet. On day two eliminate wheat and continue to eliminate sugar. On day three eliminate dairy and continue to eliminate wheat and sugar and so on.

Follow the plan closely and, by the seventh day, all seven items should have been effectively removed from your diet.

The Healthy You! Elimination Phase step-by-step meal plan begins on page 61 and accompanying recipes appear in Appendix I. Follow along exactly, or substitute one meal for another, as long as you still adhere to the elimination schedule.

Remember that the Elimination Phase is a crucial part of the program. Although you will lose weight during this segment, believe it or not, weight loss isn't the main goal. This week is really about awareness—gaining perspective on what your body has been lacking. It often takes eliminating certain foods to encourage you to make better choices. Once you reach day seven on the Elimination Phase, your diet will consist of a long list of healthy, wholesome and often natural foods that contribute to the ultimate goal of clean eating.

Elimination Phase Meal Plan

	Day 1	Day 2	Day 3	Day 4	Day 5	Day 6	Day 7
Breakfast	Healthy You! Very Berry Smoothie	Oatmeal with Fresh Berries & Milk	Healthy You! Super Green Juice	Scrambled Eggs & Oatmeal with Almond Milk	Healthy You! Radiant Red Juice	Veggie Omelet & 1/4 Melon	Spinach, Tomato & Basil Frittata with Fruit Salad
Lunch	Turkey & Avocado Sandwich	Grilled Chicken Caesar Salad	Three Bean Salad	Grilled Salmon & Citrus Salad	Vegetarian Chili	Pasta Salad	Cranberry & Quinoa Salad
Snack (optional)	Low-Fat String Cheese & Medium-Size Apple	Fat-Free, Sugar-Free Vanilla Yogurt & 10 Raw Almonds	Medium-Size Apple or Pear	Healthy You! Strawberry-Banana Smoothie	Banana & Strawberry Medley	Medium-Size Apple & 1 TBSP Peanut Butter	Vegetables & Hummus
Dinner	Grilled Herb Chicken with Steamed Broccoli and Side Salad	Chicken & Vegetable Stir-Fry over Steamed Brown Rice	Ginger-Soy Salmon with Steamed Broccoli and Brown Rice	Angel Hair Primavera	Lime-Marinated Flank Steak over Mixed Greens (6 oz glass of wine, optional)	Grilled Halibut with Tomato-Mango Salsa, Asparagus & Brown Rice (6 oz glass of wine, optional)	Chicken Soft Tacos
Eliminated items:	Sugar	Wheat (Plus Sugar)	Dairy (Plus Sugar and Wheat)	Highly Processed Foods (Plus Sugar, Wheat and Dairy)	Diet Sodas and Artificial Sweeteners (Plus Sugar, Wheat, Dairy and Highly Processed Foods)	Red Meat (Plus Sugar, Wheat, Dairy, Highly Processed Foods and Diet Sodas and Artificial Sweeteners)	Alcohol (Plus Sugar, Wheat, Dairy, Highly Processed Foods, Diet Sodas and Artificial Sweeteners and Red Meat)

Note: Detailed Elimination Phase meal plan starts on page 61 and Elimination Phase recipes can be found in Appendix I.

If you've been eating a diet comprised mainly of sugar, wheat, dairy, red meat and alcohol, you may experience some symptoms of withdrawal during the Elimination Phase. As you cut the unhealthy foods from your diet, you may feel worse before you feel better. It's common to experience headaches or strong cravings during this initial week, especially if you were consuming caffeinated soda or large amounts of sugar and alcohol before the program. Just know that these symptoms will pass and, during week two, you will find that you become more awake and energetic as you begin to feel lighter, healthier and filled with an overall greater sense of well-being. It's an incredible feeling, and any symptoms of initial withdrawal will have been worth how good you feel by the end of the program!

Learning how your body reacts to certain foods is an enlightening experience. When I first took away wheat from my diet, I was surprised to find that my frequent stomach pains disappeared. I currently eat wheat once again, but only in moderation. If I eat wheat for breakfast, I am conscious of consuming a wheat-free lunch and dinner, or vice versa. I wouldn't have known that wheat had a negative effect on my body had I not gone through the Elimination and Clean Phases of the Healthy You! program. Pay attention to how your body feels during each step of the program. You may be surprised to find that your body also performs better without sugar, wheat or dairy.

You may be asking why the Elimination Phase is so important. Let me share with you the negative impact the eliminated foods can have on your health and weight loss goals.

Day 1: Why Eliminate Sugar

According to the American Heart Association, most American adults consume 22 teaspoons of sugar a day—far more than the recommended six teaspoons for women and nine for men—and the average child consumes 32. For me, reducing my sugar intake has proved the most important dietary change and the one that has helped me best maintain a healthy body weight.

Before we continue, let me reiterate a few important points. I'm not advocating eliminating natural sugar found in fruits and some vegetables. Instead, I am asking that you reduce the non-nutritious sugar currently present in your diet. Jettison those empty calories in favor of more nutritionally beneficial foods. Natural sugar found in fruits and vegetables is acceptable, but table sugar and all items that list sugar as an ingredient—like candy, cookies, cake, pie and ice cream—should be avoided. You will find only a small amount of unrefined sugar, like honey and agavé nectar, present in a few of the recipes found in Appendix I.

Did You Know?
Refined sugar has no nutritional value and has been linked to obesity, depression, hypertension, high blood pressure, hypoglycemia, headaches, fatigue, diabetes, acne and the stiffening of arteries.

If you regularly consume sugary, non-nutritious foods like ice cream, baked goods, candy, and soda, you'll almost immediately notice positive changes when you reduce or eliminate these items.

For me, one of the most incredible benefits of cutting back on sugar was an increase in taste. As I eliminated sugar from my system, my sense of taste reemerged. I realized how delicious certain foods tasted, and I noticed that I once again appreciated the process of eating. I no longer simply jammed food down my throat; instead, I truly savored every bite, detecting subtle flavors and new aromas. It was as if my entire eating experience had been reborn.

You'll also notice that your energy level becomes more constant. You will experience fewer mid-afternoon crashes, the lethargy that often follows big meals will disappear, and you'll feel good all day long. By avoiding sugar highs and subsequent crashes, you will keep your body more in balance.

Sugar goes by many names and can often be disguised under the following:

- Corn sweetener or corn syrup
- Cane juice
- Dextrin
- Dextrose
- Fructose
- Glucose
- High-fructose corn syrup
- Lactose
- Maltodextrin
- Maltose
- Sorghum
- Sucrose
- Treacle
- Xylose

You can also find healthier, more natural sugar options such as agavé nectar, fruit juice concentrate, honey, brown rice syrup, maple syrup and molasses. Although these are good alternatives, you should still reduce or eliminate them during week one and two of the Healthy You! program.

The first step toward reducing your sugar intake is simple: pay attention to what you eat. Read labels when you're at the grocery store. Also, note that sugar isn't always listed as "sugar;" it often appears as corn syrup or high-fructose corn syrup.

People often don't realize how much sugar they consume on a regular basis. Adrianna was in her early twenties when she came to me for weight loss advice. She mentioned that she had tried everything and that, although she ate well, she still couldn't lose weight. A red flag always goes up when someone tells me they eat healthily yet experience no weight loss. So I asked Adrianna to record everything she ate over the next three days and to come back and see me.

She returned three days later with a list of everything she had consumed. She had told the truth; her meals were relatively healthy and, given what she was eating, she should have been losing rather than gaining weight. Yet I still sensed that something was off, so I dug a little deeper until Adrianna finally confessed to drinking two or three cans of soda (usually Mountain Dew) each day.

So I did some quick math for her: 165 calories per can x two cans per day x 365 days = 120,450 calories or an additional 34.4 pounds of body weight a year! 46.5 sugar grams per can x two cans per day x 365 days = 33,945 grams or almost 75 pounds of sugar a year!

Seventy-five pounds of sugar! Imagine stacking up seven 10-pound bags of sugar and then topping it off with one five-pound bag. That's how much sugar this young woman put in her body every year, and that didn't even include any other food she ate! Adrianna agreed to quit her soda habit cold turkey and, as expected, she immediately began to lose weight.

Sadly, soda is hardly the only culprit when it comes to drinking excess calories. Fancy coffee drinks, more popular today then ever, can sabotage even the most well-intentioned eater. Take into consideration that one Starbucks Grande Café Latte totals a whopping 272 calories. Consume just one a day, and you're looking at 1,904 extra calories a week or 99,008 a year. That's equivalent to 28 extra pounds annually!

Eliminating sugar and the non-nutritious empty-calorie foods made from sugar will start you on a path to healthier eating and weight loss.

Day 2: Why Eliminate Wheat

Wheat is the most common grain consumed in the American diet and, while grains can be good for you, most of us eat too much refined and processed wheat.

Did You Know?
According to the National Association of Wheat Growers, approximately 75% of all grain products in the United States are made from wheat flour.

Cardiologist and "Wheat Belly" author William Davis believes wheat to be the single largest contributor to the nationwide obesity epidemic. He says that its elimination is key to dramatic weight loss and optimal health. When you reduce or temporarily eliminate wheat from your diet, not only can this change facilitate weight loss, but you may also find that you feel better overall.

Temporarily eliminating wheat from your diet will allow you to try healthy wheat-free and gluten-free alternatives. Some of the more popular and easy to find wheat-free grains include amaranth, corn, millet, oats (gluten-free brands), rice and quinoa.

When I developed the Healthy You! program, I knew that wheat would be one of the first food items to be eliminated during week one. With two small children at home and a very hectic schedule, we were eating pasta at least once or twice a week, if not more. I enjoy pasta, but more importantly, I love how quick and simple it is to prepare. I realized it would be tough to eliminate pasta entirely from our diet, so instead, I made the simple switch from regular to rice pasta. My husband hardly even noticed the change, but both of us did notice that we felt better after eating rice pasta than the usual wheat-based version.

Another reason to give up wheat is that more and more people are discovering that they suffer from wheat or gluten intolerances or sensitivities. Sensitivity to wheat can cause headaches, weight gain, brain fog and abdominal pain or discomfort.

A wheat allergy differs from a gluten sensitivity; if you have a wheat allergy, your body might react to several different components found in wheat. (There are more than two dozen potential wheat allergens of which gluten is just one.) Gluten intolerance or celiac disease occurs, however, when the digestive system cannot tolerate gluten.

People often use gluten and wheat interchangeably; yet, gluten is not wheat. Gluten is a protein found in wheat, rye and barley. Gluten often gives foods their chewy texture. Bread flours typically contain the highest amounts of gluten.

Did You Know?
The U.S. Food and Drug Administration identifies wheat as one of eight foods (along with cow's milk, eggs, peanuts, tree nuts, fish, shellfish and soybeans) that cause 90% of food-related allergic reactions.

Use the Elimination Phase as a way to determine whether a wheat-free diet works for you. If you don't notice a difference in how you feel, you can reintroduce healthy whole wheat products to your diet after the two-week period—but healthy is the key term here.

Day 3: Why Eliminate Dairy

Dairy refers to milk and any products made from milk such as cheese, yogurt, ice cream, cream and butter. Chances are, you've seen the clever "Got Milk?" campaign. More than 90% of all Americans are familiar with the ads, making them part of one of the most famous campaigns in advertising history. The ad series started in 1993 as part of an attempt by the California Milk Processor Board to stop the declining sales of milk and was later licensed to the National Milk Processor Board. In 2002, USA Today named the campaign one of the ten best commercials of all time! The campaign worked; studies confirmed that people were indeed drinking milk more often.

The "dairy is good for you" versus "dairy is bad for you" debate has raged for decades. There are those who believe in all the benefits touted by the Milk Board. However, others feel that all the advertising encourages people to drink something that we shouldn't consume in the first place. In fact, in 2012 the Physicians Committee for Responsible Medicine petitioned the U.S. Department of Agriculture to remove milk from school lunches. Research showed that not only did dairy not improve bone health, but that it also acted as the number one source of saturated fat in children's diets and could increase childhood obesity.

The reason for such a strong debate? Science has not yet reached a firm conclusion on the advantages and disadvantages of drinking milk.

So where do I stand on milk and dairy products, you ask? I grew up regularly drinking milk, and my three-and five-year-old children still drink organic milk before school and after dinner. But as they get older, I have slowly cut back on the amount of milk they consume. Personally, I can't remember the last time I drank a glass of milk. These days I only consume dairy when I'm having a treat like an occasional ice cream cone, some cheese or a yogurt. And instead of cow's milk, I now use substitutes like almond milk (my favorite) or rice milk.

I'm not against eating dairy per se, yet when I first reduced my milk consumption, I noticed a few immediate, positive results. My skin cleared up, I no longer suffered from as many sinus problems, and I immediately lost weight.

As is the case with the consumption of processed foods, sugar and so on, I believe that moderation is always best. The Healthy You! program allows you to determine what eliminating dairy does for your body. If you currently consume a large amount of milk (or products containing milk like cheese, yogurt and baked goods), you may also notice some immediate, positive results when eliminating dairy. Should you decide to bring dairy back following the program, you'll be better prepared to make wise choices.

Reducing my milk consumption really made a difference in how I felt and with my weight loss success. In the end, of course, it's up to you whether you reduce or eliminate dairy from your diet. Yet most people who have done the Healthy You! program report feeling an almost immediate difference upon giving up dairy. I think you'll notice the benefits, too.

Did you know?

Eggs are often categorized as "dairy" when, in fact, they are not. Dairy is defined as a product or by-product coming from the mammary gland of a mammal. Milk, cheese, and yogurt, are all dairy products. However, eggs do not come from the mammary gland of a mammal; therefore, they are not dairy.

Day 4: Why Eliminate Processed Foods

Until the 20th century, hardly any foods were processed. These days, even a quick walk through the supermarket shows how greatly times have changed. In fact, for many people, processed foods comprise the majority of their daily caloric intake and research shows Americans spend nearly 90% of their food budget on processed foods!

So what exactly defines processed foods? These are foods no longer appearing in their natural state and often packaged for convenience.

Processed foods contain a host of empty calories in the form of sugar and fat. In today's fast-paced world, convenience is often prized over nutritional value, and processed food can seem a simple and quick solution. These foods may provide calories, but not the nutrients we need to support a healthy, balanced diet.

Some common processed food offenders include:
- Chips, pretzels and most packaged snack foods
- Fast food
- Pre-packaged or ready-made meals
- Canned foods (the worst offenders contain several ingredients aside from the main ingredient)
- White bread
- Hot dogs, sausages, packaged lunch meats

Processed foods also contain large amounts of added salt (sodium). According to the Mayo Clinic, "Salt is added to make food more flavorful. Salt makes soups thicker, reduces dryness in crackers and pretzels and increases sweetness in cakes and cookies. Salt also helps disguise a metallic or chemical aftertaste in products such as soft drinks."

Although it might be difficult to eliminate all processed foods, try to eliminate as many as possible. You may notice that some of the Healthy You! recipes like vegetarian chili and vegetable soup include canned beans rather than dried beans. Although I believe that dried would be better than canned, I acknowledge that canned beans are much more convenient. Soaking and cooking a large batch of beans can be very time consuming and might not be realistic when factoring in a busy schedule. If you do choose canned beans, try to select organic brands that don't contain any additional ingredients.

Eliminating most processed foods will compel you to make more intelligent and healthy food choices. Most people choose fast food because of its convenience. Just a few minutes in the drive-through can lead to lunch or dinner for you and the entire family. When preparing your own meals at home, you may have to factor in an additional 15 minutes or so, but the end result—a thinner, healthier, happier you—will be undoubtedly worth it. So instead of frequenting the local fast food spot, stop by the market. Pick up some chicken, vegetables and rice. I can cook a stir-fry chicken dish in less than 30 minutes. It tastes delicious and, as a bonus, every time I prepare the dish, I know that I have taken a step toward better health.

Looking for an even quicker option? Most grocery stores now offer ready-to-eat grilled chicken roasters, bag salads and pre-washed and cut microwaveable vegetables.

No matter how hectic your life may be, know that alternatives to fast food and junk food do exist. Before my children were born and I traveled constantly, I had to make good food choices while running airport-to-airport, hotel-to-hotel and meeting-to-meeting. The secret to success stemmed from having the discipline to choose healthy food over processed food.

Reducing or eliminating packaged foods and increasing foods sold in their natural state will help reduce your intake of processed foods. If you do choose to incorporate some processed foods back into your diet after the 14 days, being conscious of ingredients can help you make better choices. If you haven't spent much time studying nutrition labels, you may be amazed at what you find. I still remember when I first took notice of nutritional information and ingredients charts. I was amazed to find that some ice cream brands listed 20 or more ingredients—many of which I couldn't even pronounce. I love ice cream and enjoy it on occasion as a treat, but I now look for brands that use only a few ingredients—all words I can easily pronounce like cream, milk and sugar. I now skip brands that list such items as dried cane syrup, butter, sodium bicarbonate, carrageenan, guar gum and sunflower oil.

Rest assured that this doesn't mean you can't ever again indulge in processed foods like a bag of chips or a candy bar; it just means that you should enjoy those foods as special treats and not as diet staples.

Day 5: Why Eliminate Diet Soda and Artificial Sweeteners

Many people believe they are doing themselves (and their weight) a favor by using artificial sweeteners or drinking diet soda. But artificial sweeteners and diet sodas may actually work against you in the battle of the bulge. According to Dr. David Ludwig, an obesity and weight loss specialist at the Harvard-affiliated Boston Children's Hospital, people may be more likely to replace the calories they're saving by using artificial sweeteners with other calories, ultimately offsetting any weight loss benefits. He also says that artificial sweeteners over stimulate our sugar receptors and may change the way we taste food—making healthy foods less appealing and even making us crave sweet foods.

> **Did You Know?**
> A study published by the American Academy of Neurology suggests that people who drink more than four cans of soda per day are 30% more likely to suffer from depression than those who don't drink any, and the risk is even greater for those who consume diet sodas.

In fact, a study in the Journal of Behavioral Neuroscience shows that artificial sweeteners, which people often believe help prevent weight gain, actually induce hormonal and physiological responses that can have the opposite effect. The study used two groups of rats. One group was fed sugar-sweetened yogurt, while the other was given yogurt sweetened with saccharin, a commonly used artificial sweetener. Scientists found that the artificial sweeteners stimulated the rats' appetites and made them eat more. The rats given the artificial sweetener not only gained weight and increased their body fat percentages, but the group also experienced a decrease in core body temperatures, which slowed down their metabolisms.

Again, moderation is key. Like most people, I enjoy a diet soda every now and then, but I usually limit my consumption to one can per week. The thing I noticed most when I eliminated both sugar and artificial sweeteners from my diet was how much better I could taste my foods. Foods that once tasted bland now exploded with flavor. Finding healthy food more pleasing to the taste buds made it easier to make smart choices and, consequently, to lose weight.

Day 6: Why Eliminate Red Meat

I enjoy a good steak every now and then, but we've all heard the supposed correlation between red meat consumption and heart disease. In fact, an AARP study by the National Institutes of Health tested more than 500,000 Americans and showed that people who ate the most red or processed meat over a 10-year period were likely to die sooner than those who consumed less.

Marki McCullouth, PhD, a nutritional epidemiologist with the American Cancer Society says, "The association between consumption of red and processed meats and cancer, particularly colorectal cancer, is very consistent."

I'm 45, and like many people my age, I grew up eating red meat on a daily basis. Ground beef, hot dogs, beef tacos, beef burritos, hamburgers, steaks and beef stews were just a few of the meals my mom regularly prepared. If our dinner didn't contain beef, my dad didn't consider it a real meal.

It wasn't until I went away to college that I questioned eating meat. I lived in the dorms during my freshman year and felt disgusted by the meat served in the cafeteria—most didn't resemble the meat dishes I had grown up eating. Although I continued to eat some chicken and fish, I stopped eating red meat completely for nearly 10 years. It wasn't until I entered graduate school and met my husband that I decided to give it another try.

One night at dinner, my husband ordered a filet mignon. I'm not sure what got into me, but his steak looked and smelled very appealing. I remember asking if I could try a bite. At first he assumed I was kidding, but he finally agreed. I only had two bites of his steak that night, but consuming meat after a decade was a big deal for me. I still don't eat a lot of red meat, but since that night, I no longer steer clear altogether. I consume red meat about once every week or two, and I make sure to always order a lean cut. One of my favorite meals—typically enjoyed only once a month—consists of filet mignon, French fries or mashed potatoes and a good glass of red wine.

I believe that red meat can be part of a healthy diet as long as you select lean cuts and keep the serving size moderate. Red meat consumption only becomes problematic when eaten too often and in large quantities. After creating the Healthy You! program, I've seen that you can eat a small amount of red meat once a week and still continue to lose weight.

Did You Know?
The USDA defines a lean cut of beef as a 3.5-ounce serving with less than 10 grams of fat and an extra-lean cut of beef as a 3.5-ounce serving with less than five grams of fat. Your typical restaurant steak measures six to 12 ounces and can weigh as much as 20 ounces!

On the Healthy You! program, you will eliminate red meat toward the end of week one and throughout the entire second week. After the two weeks end, should you decide to incorporate red meat back into your diet, choose cuts with the least amount of fat such as sirloin, tenderloin (filet mignon) or T-bone, and keep the serving size to three to four ounces for women and four to six ounces for men. I suggest eating red meat no more frequently than once a week.

Day 7: Why Eliminate Alcohol

According to Betty Kovacs, Director of Nutrition for the New York Obesity Research Center Weight Loss Program, alcohol consumption can cause you to eat more and, therefore, to gain weight. In fact, research shows that people ingest 20% more calories when alcohol is consumed before a meal—and 33% more if you also include the alcohol's caloric total.

Although I admittedly enjoy a couple drinks on the weekends or the occasional nice glass of wine with my husband, it is undeniable that eliminating or reducing alcohol makes the weight loss process much easier.

We often associate only food with calories and forget that beverages can also be highly caloric. According to the National Center for Health Statistics, regular consumers of alcoholic beverages can get as many as 16% of their total daily calories from alcohol.

Calories from alcohol quickly add up, especially when mixed drinks are on your menu. Find below a partial list of popular cocktails and their (high) caloric averages:

Margarita	550 Calories
Mai Tai	620 Calories
Piña Colada	586 Calories
Mud Slide	556 Calories

When watching your weight, it's best to skip the fancy drinks and stick to beer, wine or drinks mixed with non-caloric mixers like club soda. A typical 12-ounce beer contains approximately 150 calories, a five-ounce glass of wine approximately 120 and a one-and-a-half-ounce shot of liquor approximately 100. Making careful selections can help ward off additional calories, which later translate to extra pounds.

Did You Know?
One 10-ounce Long Island Iced Tea contains about the same number of calories as a McDonald's Big Mac!

If you are trying to lose weight, be smart about your alcohol consumption. Save the alcohol for special occasions, or drink only once a week after you've completed the Healthy You! program. Once you attain your weight loss goal, you should be able to drink alcohol in moderation without gaining back the pounds you've shed. When it comes to alcohol, moderation is key!

CHAPTER 8

The Clean Phase

The Clean Phase is a seven-day continuation of the final day of the Elimination Phase. During the Clean Phase, you will continue to eat a diet free of sugar, wheat, dairy, processed foods, diet soda and artificial sweeteners, red meat and alcohol.

To some, the Clean Phase may seem a little extreme, but remember that this period is temporary and will help you obtain immediate results. During this phase, your body will start to feel lighter as excess weight comes off. Although this will likely prove the most challenging week, it will also be the most rewarding.

This phase depends upon clean eating. You will select foods that are fresh, wholesome and nutrient-rich while also free from artificial ingredients and preservatives. You will also experiment with new fruits, vegetables, nuts, seeds and legumes. During this phase, your body should start to feel rejuvenated.

Both the Elimination Phase and the Clean Phase are absolutely crucial. These two weeks will help you reevaluate what you've been eating out of habit. Especially for those individuals who tend to put a lot of empty (non-nutritional) calories into their bodies or eat a lot of prepackaged and processed food, these two weeks will prove eye-opening.

You may have suffered some symptoms of withdrawal during the Elimination Phase, but the Clean Phase focuses on nourishing your body. You should begin to feel more balanced and alive. Your thoughts may become more clear and focused. This week means taking care of your body and giving it what it needs. You will likely feel more vibrant and energetic as you reach the end of the clean week. The Clean Phase can forever change the way you think about food, making you a more mindful eater.

Even once you reach your goal weight, you may still fall off track at times. When a family vacation, a cruise or an especially stressful work week causes me to pack on a few unwanted pounds, spending just one week on the Clean Phase gets me back to a healthy eating program that helps drop that excess weight.

Week 2: The Clean Phase (Days 8-14)

Continue to eliminate sugar, wheat, dairy, highly processed foods, diet soda and artificial sweeteners, red meat and alcohol.

Find the Healthy You! Clean Phase meal plan in the chart below. As previously mentioned, you can follow the program precisely or substitute one meal for another. If you really enjoy one of the meals, you can choose to have it more than once. If there is a meal that you don't particularly care for, you can remove it from the plan and substitute it with a meal from another day. A detailed, step-by-step meal plan begins on page 69 and complementary recipes for the Clean Phase can be found in Appendix I.

Clean Phase Meal Plan

	Day 8	Day 9	Day 10	Day 11	Day 12	Day 13	Day 14
Breakfast	Healthy You! Super Green Juice	Healthy You! Pineapple-Avocado Smoothie	Healthy You! Strawberry-Banana Smoothie	Veggie Scramble & Oatmeal	Healthy You! Radiant Red Juice	Veggie Omelet and Fresh Fruit Cup	Healthy You! Super Green Juice
Lunch	Grilled Chicken & Chickpea Garden Salad	Vegetable Soup & Salad	Lentil Salad	Walnut & Pear Salad	Greek Salad with Grilled Chicken	Wild Rice & Spinach Soup	Crab, Mango & Avocado Stack
Snack (optional)	Tortilla Chips & Fresh Salsa	Celery & 1 TBSP Peanut Butter	Small Handful Red or Green Grapes	Healthy You! Magic Mango Smoothie	Medium-Size Apple & 10 Raw Almonds	Vegetables & Hummus	Medium-Size Apple or Pear
Dinner	Crab Cakes & Green Beans	Black Bean Tostadas	Agavé Rosemary Chicken & Wild Rice	Fish Tacos with Mango-Avocado Salsa	California Roll (Sushi) with Edamame	Mushroom Risotto	Fish in Parchment with Pineapple-Mango Chutney, Basmati Rice and Asparagus
Eliminated items:	Sugar, Wheat, Dairy, Highly Processed Foods, Diet Soda and Artificial Sweeteners, Red Meat and Alcohol	Sugar, Wheat, Dairy, Highly Processed Foods, Diet Soda and Artificial Sweeteners, Red Meat and Alcohol	Sugar, Wheat, Dairy, Highly Processed Foods, Diet Soda and Artificial Sweeteners, Red Meat and Alcohol	Sugar, Wheat, Dairy, Highly Processed Foods, Diet Soda and Artificial Sweeteners, Red Meat and Alcohol	Sugar, Wheat, Dairy, Highly Processed Foods, Diet Soda and Artificial Sweeteners, Red Meat and Alcohol	Sugar, Wheat, Dairy, Highly Processed Foods, Diet Soda and Artificial Sweeteners, Red Meat and Alcohol	Sugar, Wheat, Dairy, Highly Processed Foods, Diet Soda and Artificial Sweeteners, Red Meat and Alcohol

Note: Detailed Clean Phase meal plan starts on page 69 and Clean Phase recipes can be found in Appendix I.

Healthy You! Program Recap:

Week 1: Elimination

Day 1: Eliminate Sugar

Day 2: Eliminate Wheat (Plus Sugar)

Day 3: Eliminate Dairy (Plus Sugar and Wheat)

Day 4: Eliminate Highly Processed Foods (Plus Sugar, Wheat and Dairy)

Day 5: Eliminate Diet Soda and Artificial Sweeteners (Plus Sugar, Wheat, Dairy and Highly Processed Foods)

Day 6: Eliminate Red Meat (Plus Sugar, Wheat, Dairy, Highly Processed Foods and Diet Soda and Artificial Sweeteners)

Day 7: Eliminate Alcohol (Plus Sugar, Wheat, Dairy, Highly Processed Foods, Diet Soda and Artificial Sweeteners and Red Meat)

Week 2: Clean

Days 8-14: Eliminate Sugar, Wheat, Dairy, Highly Processed Foods, Diet Soda and Artificial Sweeteners, Red Meat and Alcohol

CHAPTER 9

Healthy You! Meal Plan

I've learned that when following a weight loss program, "simple" is always key. Although some of us enjoy preparing elaborate meals, they aren't always conducive to time constraints and extremely busy schedules. For that reason, the Healthy You! program offers meals that are simple to make and easy to find at most any restaurant.

As mentioned earlier, the meal plan is meant to be flexible. As long as the meal adheres to the program i.e. no dairy once dairy is eliminated, no red meat once red meat is eliminated, etc. you can feel free to substitute one meal for another. You can also choose to eat the same meal more than once or choose to select another meal if the scheduled meal isn't something you care for.

Some people like to be told exactly what to eat on a weight loss program, while others want more flexibility. Personally, I've never been able to follow a strict menu plan. What if I was unable to have cedar plank salmon and grilled asparagus on Tuesday for lunch? I happen to love these foods, but the reality is that I may not have been in a position to make or order that exact meal that day.

However, if you prefer structure and a program that dictates every meal, follow the weekly meal plan. You'll know exactly what to eat for breakfast, lunch, snack and dinner throughout the entire 14-day Healthy You! program.

When I've attempted diets in the past, I've typically strayed from the plan after three to five days because I didn't like all the menu items, and no substitutions were offered. Some programs would entail in-depth recipes for all three meals. And although I undoubtedly enjoy a home-cooked, healthy meal, I don't have time to prepare breakfast, lunch and dinner from scratch every single day. The HealthyYou! weight loss program allows you to spend as much or as little time on meal preparation as your schedule allows. You're the boss; the plan just provides suggested guidelines to follow.

If you don't like fish, simply select a Healthy You! approved chicken or vegetarian recipe instead. Don't have time to cook lunch and dinner? Make an extra serving of three-bean salad one evening, and also eat it for lunch the next day. Have plans to go out for lunch or dinner? Many of the menu items can be ordered at your favorite restaurant. The plan has been developed to work with your schedule and your active, mobile lifestyle.

The following pages include your step-by-step meal plan for both the Elimination Phase and the Clean Phase. Detailed recipes for every meal can be found in Appendix I.

Elimination Phase Meal Plan

DAY 1

BREAKFAST

Healthy You! Very Berry Smoothie

LUNCH

Turkey and Avocado Sandwich

SNACK

Low-Fat String Cheese (approximately 1 oz or one snack-size serving)

Medium-Size Apple or Other Piece of Fresh Fruit

DINNER

Grilled Herb Chicken with Steamed Broccoli and Side Salad

NOTE: Eliminate Sugar

DAY 2

BREAKFAST

Oatmeal with Fresh Berries and Milk

LUNCH

Grilled Chicken Caesar Salad

SNACK

Fat-Free, Sugar-Free Vanilla Yogurt and 10 Raw Almonds

DINNER

Chicken and Vegetable Stir-Fry over Steamed Brown Rice

NOTE: Eliminate Sugar and Wheat

DAY 3

BREAKFAST
Healthy You! Super Green Juice

LUNCH
Three Bean Salad

SNACK
Medium-Size Apple or Pear

DINNER
Ginger-Soy Salmon with Steamed Broccoli and Brown Rice

NOTE: Eliminate Sugar, Wheat and Dairy

DAY 4

BREAKFAST
Scrambled Eggs and Oatmeal with Almond Milk

LUNCH
Grilled Salmon and Citrus Salad

SNACK
HealthyYou! Strawberry-Banana Smoothie

DINNER
Angel Hair Primavera

NOTE: Eliminate Sugar, Wheat, Dairy and Highly Processed Foods

DAY 5

BREAKFAST
Healthy You! Radiant Red Juice

LUNCH
Vegetarian Chili

SNACK
Banana and Strawberry Medley

DINNER
Lime-Marinated Flank Steak over Mixed Greens

OPTIONAL
One 6 oz Glass of Wine

NOTE: Eliminate Sugar, Wheat, Dairy, Highly Processed Foods and Diet Soda and Artificial Sweeteners

DAY 6

BREAKFAST

Veggie Omelet and ¼ Melon

LUNCH

Pasta Salad

SNACK

Medium-Size Apple and 1 Tablespoon Natural Peanut Butter

DINNER

Grilled Halibut with Fresh Tomato-Mango Salsa with
Steamed Asparagus and Brown Rice

OPTIONAL

One 6 oz Glass of Wine

*NOTE: Eliminate Sugar, Wheat, Dairy and Highly Processed Foods, Diet Soda
and Artificial Sweeteners and Red Meat*

DAY 7

BREAKFAST
Spinach, Tomato and Basil Frittata with Fresh Fruit Salad

LUNCH
Cranberry and Quinoa Salad

SNACK
Vegetables and Hummus

DINNER
Chicken Soft Tacos

NOTE: Eliminate Sugar, Wheat, Dairy and Highly Processed Foods, Diet Soda and Artificial Sweeteners, Red Meat and Alcohol

Clean Phase Meal Plan

DAY 8

BREAKFAST
Healthy You! Super Green Juice

LUNCH
Grilled Chicken and Chickpea Garden Salad

SNACK
Tortilla Chips and Fresh Salsa

DINNER
Crab Cakes and Green Beans

NOTE: Eliminate Sugar, Wheat, Dairy and Highly Processed Foods, Diet Soda and Artificial Sweeteners, Red Meat and Alcohol

DAY 9

BREAKFAST

Healthy You! Pineapple-Avocado Smoothie

LUNCH

Vegetable Soup and Salad

SNACK

Celery and 1 Tablespoon Natural Peanut Butter

DINNER

Black Bean Tostadas

NOTE: Eliminate Sugar, Wheat, Dairy and Highly Processed Foods, Diet Soda and Artificial Sweeteners, Red Meat and Alcohol

DAY 10

BREAKFAST

Healthy You! Strawberry-Banana Smoothie

LUNCH

Lentil Salad

SNACK

Small Handful Red or Green Grapes

DINNER

Agavé Rosemary Chicken and Wild Rice

NOTE: Eliminate Sugar, Wheat, Dairy and Highly Processed Foods, Diet Soda and Artificial Sweeteners, Red Meat and Alcohol

DAY 11

BREAKFAST

Veggie Scramble and Oatmeal

LUNCH

Walnut and Pear Salad

SNACK

Healthy You! Mango Smoothie

DINNER

Fish Tacos with Mango-Avocado Salsa

NOTE: Eliminate Sugar, Wheat, Dairy and Highly Processed Foods, Diet Soda and Artificial Sweeteners, Red Meat and Alcohol

DAY 12

BREAKFAST
Healthy You! Radiant Red Juice

LUNCH
Greek Salad with Grilled Chicken

SNACK
Medium-Size Apple and 10 Raw Almonds

DINNER
California Roll (Sushi) with Edamame

NOTE: Eliminate Sugar, Wheat, Dairy and Highly Processed Foods, Diet Soda and Artificial Sweeteners, Red Meat and Alcohol

DAY 13

BREAKFAST

Veggie Omelet and Fresh Fruit Cup

LUNCH

Wild Rice and Spinach Soup

SNACK

Vegetables and Hummus

DINNER

Mushroom Risotto

NOTE: Eliminate Sugar, Wheat, Dairy and Highly Processed Foods, Diet Soda and Artificial Sweeteners, Red Meat and Alcohol

DAY 14

BREAKFAST
Healthy You! Super Green Juice

LUNCH
Crab, Mango and Avocado Stack

SNACK
Medium-Size Apple or Pear

DINNER
Fish in Parchment with Pineapple-Mango Chutney, Basmati Rice and Asparagus

NOTE: Eliminate Sugar, Wheat, Dairy and Highly Processed Foods, Diet Soda and Artificial Sweeteners, Red Meat and Alcohol

PART THREE

Ensure Your Success

CHAPTER 10

Remove Your Trigger Foods

I know it's not always easy to change familiar eating habits. Most of us have a few foods that always seem to sabotage our diets. For me, it's anything containing chocolate, but my mom can't resist anything salty. I've learned from trial and error—some big errors, might I add—about how to cope with my trigger foods and prevent them from ruining my well-intentioned habits.

Years ago, I read that the best way to regain self-control with a certain food was to keep an abundance in the house. The theory claimed that if you had several packages readily available and didn't declare any food forbidden, then you wouldn't feel like you had to eat the entire portion in one sitting (since there would be more at your disposal to eat at any time). So I decided to give it a try.

The concept seemed to make sense, and the article touched precisely on the reason I often consumed an entire box at once. I always planned to start living healthily "tomorrow," so I thought I had to overindulge before enforcing those limitations. To test the theory, I went out and bought three boxes of Double Stuf Oreos.

That night I enjoyed a few cookies before putting the first package back in the cupboard next to the other two. Immediately I thought, "Wow, this really works." Yet a few minutes later, I returned to the cupboard for a couple cookies and then again for a few more. Before I knew it, I had finished the first bag and gotten into the next. I felt sick and utterly disgusted with myself. So much for their theory, I thought; it may work for some, but it definitely didn't work for me. Over the years, I've tried this system several more times—each time with a different trigger food—and I always end up regretting the decision.

My philosophy on trigger foods is the following: if they're around, you're going to eat them. If they're not around, you won't. That doesn't mean you have to give up your favorite foods altogether; it just means that you should reserve them for special occasions and purchase them in moderation. Removing your trigger foods during the 14-day HealthyYou! program will set you up for sustainable success.

Did You Know?

Multiple studies performed by Brian Wansink, author of "Mindless Eating" and former executive director of the USDA's Center for Nutrition Policy and Promotion, found that visible foods trigger eating. In fact, one study conducted with Hershey's Kisses found that candies placed in clear jars were consumed 46% more quickly than those placed in opaque jars.

To start, you need to determine which foods trigger you to overeat. For example, I can keep a gallon of my favorite ice cream in the freezer for months without overindulging; I simply enjoy a scoop when I feel like it. But I can't keep a bag of chocolate candies or chocolate chip cookies in the house without losing control. My husband's trigger foods are pretzels, potato chips and cheese. For my mom, it's peanuts. For my sister, it's pasta (she'll indulge until she feels sick).

Once you've determined which unhealthy foods prompt you to overeat, remove them from your kitchen. You can bring them back into your house once you've spent 14 days on the Healthy You! program. You'll be amazed at how two weeks spent improving your eating habits can permanently alter the foods you crave and your ability to make better choices.

The HealthyYou! program ultimately helped me gain control over my trigger foods. While working as a management consultant after graduate school, I had been assigned to a yearlong project at Nestlé. I was excited to be working at a consumer products company and especially thrilled since Nestlé produces some of my favorite foods. I soon realized, however, that the project—although good for my career—wasn't going to be good for my waistline.

Most recognize Nestlé as the manufacturer of some of the most popular chocolate products in the world. What you may not know, though, is that Nestlé also makes promotional items for some of the top Hollywood movies. I worked at Nestlé about four days a week and, on many days, I would find one of those promotional items, usually a chocolate-themed representation of the movie it advertised, on my desk when I arrived in the morning. Given that chocolate is probably my biggest trigger food, I of course happily indulged.

Within just a few weeks of working on the project, I gained more than 10 pounds and felt awful. Since I hadn't yet developed the HealthyYou! program, instead of selecting my favorite promotional items and discarding or giving away the rest, I ate every single one gifted to me. Every night before bed, I swore that "tomorrow" I would start eating mindfully. The problem? "Tomorrow" never came. Every day replayed the same story: I would overindulge on chocolate, feel horrible, gain even more weight and promise to change my ways. The cycle lasted until the project finished, but that didn't mark the end of my problem with trigger foods.

While working as the senior vice president of operations for The Active Sports Network, better known as Active.com, I had a similar experience. Two of my favorite coworkers always kept a large glass jar in their offices filled with chocolate. As you can imagine, I visited their offices regularly to get my chocolate fix. One day I entered the office and, about to pop off the lid, noticed a note on top that read:"Dawna, Keep Out!"

You know you have a problem when your colleagues are comfortable telling their boss to"Keep Out!"Today, I'd be able to walk by the jar and not think much about it. But before doing the HealthyYou! program, it was a struggle to stay away.

Acknowledge which foods you tend to overeat, and take them out of your house and office during the 14-day Healthy You! program. You can incorporate these foods back into your diet after the two weeks, as no foods are permanently banned. The program helped me learn how to enjoy my favorite foods in moderation, and it can help you do the same.

List the three or four unhealthy foods that trigger you to overeat—foods that always seem to sabotage your healthy eating intentions or weight loss goals.

1. _____

2. _____

3. _____

4. _____

Then remove these trigger foods from your kitchen and/or office for at least the next 14 days.

CHAPTER 11

Find a Support Team

I had the opportunity to meet Richard Simmons during a taping of the "MARTHA" show. Although I've always thought Richard was a bit quirky, I admire him for helping so many people take the first step toward positive body change.

Richard may not have the "perfect" lean, muscular male body worshiped by so many in Hollywood, but when I met him, I could immediately sense how comfortable he felt with his body. It was refreshing to witness someone so content in his own skin, and his uninhibited energy proved contagious.

I could easily see why so many men and women achieve their weight loss goals with Richard as their cheerleader. You may not be lucky enough to have a celebrity guru personally support you, but make sure you do have a few positive and energetic supporters who can provide encouragement throughout your journey.

Did You Know?

People who come together as a team to lose weight significantly influence one another's weight loss and can achieve similar results. A study published in 2012 by the Miriam Hospital Weight Control and Diabetes Center suggests that working together can increase your odds of achieving significant weight loss by 20%.

Try to find a friend, family member or co-worker to do the program with you. Over the holidays, my husband and I both gained a few extra pounds. Although I only gained three or four pounds, the excess sugar and alcohol I consumed during the month of December left me feeling sluggish and heavy. My husband and I decided to tackle the Healthy You! program together. Doing it as a team made it so much more fun. We were able to plan special dinners with one another and even made it a point to visit restaurants that offered Healthy You!-approved meals like grilled mahi mahi with fresh mango salsa. We dined at our favorite sushi restaurant and relished the perfect date night, without going off the program.

Within a week, I was back to my pre-holiday weight and had returned to my normal eating habits, which almost always consist of a balance of healthy eating and occasional indulgences. My husband lost nearly 10 pounds in the first 10 days of the program, and he was thrilled to comfortably fit back into his dress pants again.

Doing the program together made it that much easier to stay motivated. Whether you enlist one other person to also do the program or gather a larger group, it doesn't matter. I've found that having one partner (or many) on the program can fast-track your success.

My friend's mom Mary is a great example of someone who used a large group for inspiration to stick to a healthy eating program. Mary's company employs more than 100 people, and once or twice a year, the company hosts a corporate challenge to encourage good eating and exercise habits. The 12-week, team-based challenge wasn't something Mary thought she'd enjoy, although she felt inspired by the thought of losing weight. Mary explains, "I did not appreciate the team factor until I got started with the challenge. It wasn't until I was assigned to a team that it really hit me how important my contribution was to the team's success." Mary says she was motivated by the support of the team as well as the accountability she felt. As Mary began to lose weight and witness changes in her body, she became even more motivated. She says,"This challenge worked because being part of a group with similar goals kept me motivated, and the extra motivation equaled more weight loss."

If you don't have a formal support team like Mary did, you can take advantage of several online options. Simply sharing your story online can garner all the support you need. Just following a fitness blog or commenting on related posts can keep you motivated. Also make sure that your family and friends know you're on the program. The extra support you'll receive from them can really pay off.

Ask Dawna

It's hard to stay motivated when my husband continually tells me I'm fat. What can I do to make him stop?

I usually tell people to avoid anyone who acts as a negative influence or makes you feel worse about yourself. But in this case, I can't tell you to avoid your husband. Instead, you do need to confront him. If you're unhappy with the way you look, tell him that you too are not satisfied with your body and that you plan to start fresh and to make some positive and measurable changes. Let him know that this is going to be difficult for you; you will need his support. Be specific, and let him know how hurtful it is to hear that he's so dissatisfied with your body. Let him know that even small pats on the back can be helpful. Seemingly insignificant remarks like,"I'm proud of you for going on a walk!" and "Great job opting for the fruit instead of fries!" will help carry you through to the next day.

Also consider asking your husband to join you in your commitment to eat better and be more active. It's much easier to stick with change when you have a support system. Enlisting a partner will make the journey more fun and allow you to make positive changes as a couple.

People are heading online in droves to read about or share their weight loss stories. I met one such woman, Callie, at last year's Women's Half Marathon. Callie has two children under the age of two and really wanted to get back in shape after her pregnancies. She found that blogging about her journey to become healthier kept her motivated. According to Callie, "Accountability is key when working toward a healthier lifestyle. Over the years, I've learned that accountability can be found in the most unexpected places. For me, that place was from total strangers on the Internet." Callie started sharing her story on her blog, and she quickly found a community that celebrated her accomplishments with her, provided encouragement in tough times and held her accountable when she strayed from her goals. Callie says, "Finding a community of support online inspires me to achieve my goals."

Support can come in many different forms. If you can't find a friend or co-worker with whom to join forces, simply keeping a journal or a blog, much like Callie's, can provide the support and accountability you need.

The ideal support team:
- Wants to see you succeed
- Is positive and energetic
- Provides constant praise
- Has your best interest at heart
- Shares similar goals
- Can be found in unexpected places like on the Internet

CHAPTER 12

Track Your Progress

When embarking on a weight loss plan, people have mixed opinions on how often you should weigh yourself. Depending on where you are in your journey, the scale can be your best friend or your worst enemy. For most, the scale has emotional consequences. When the scale shows you a number you want to see, you're filled with joy, but when it shows you a number that's not so great, you may experience despair and self-loathing. It's funny how a little piece of plastic can have such a profound effect on one's mood.

After years of a love-hate relationship with my scale, I finally realized that it can serve as an ally in my quest for weight management. But first, I had to learn how to make friends with the machine.

We've all heard the advice on popular talk shows and in best-selling diet books to simply throw out one's scale. Although it may sound liberating, it's not the way to win the weight loss battle. The scale is a necessary tool to help you achieve your goals. Don't worry; this doesn't mean you'll be weighing yourself every day for the rest of your life. But I do encourage you to weigh yourself sporadically during the 14-day HealthyYou! program and then daily once you reach your ideal weight. Once you meet your goal, weighing yourself every day can help you understand the normal ebb and flow of your own body, helping you to stay on track.

I know many people who don't believe in weighing themselves regularly. But when they do finally step on a scale—whether in a doctor's office or at a friend's house—they can't believe their eyes. "How did I gain those 10, 15, 20 pounds?" they ask incredulously. Had they only viewed the scale as their ally and used it consistently as a motivational tool, they would have been able to heed the weight gain warning much sooner.

I know from weighing myself daily that I can overindulge for a night or two and still maintain my ideal weight. But I've also learned that any longer than two days in a row of unhealthy eating, and the scale will reflect a gain.

Weigh yourself the morning before you start the Healthy You! program, and write down your starting figure. Don't weigh yourself during the first week of the program, but weigh yourself again on the morning of the eighth day—once you've completed an entire week on the program (unless otherwise specified in the "Who Are You" chapter). Remember that everyone is different. I lost four pounds during week one, and my husband lost eight. I have worked with others who have lost as few as three and as many as ten-plus.

Starting on the eighth day, weigh yourself every other day. Remember that weight fluctuations can occur for many reasons including sodium consumption, your menstrual cycles, dehydration and late night eating. Record your progress, and refer to it often.

While it's true that the scale can be an important tool in weight management, it's important to remember that it doesn't always reveal the whole story. If you've been sedentary but then embark on a weight loss and exercise program simultaneously—the best way to achieve and sustain weight loss—then the scale may not tell you everything you want to know. Muscle weighs more than fat, so it's possible to drastically change the way your body looks and not see the number you'd hoped for on the scale.

To get a true indication of how your body responds to diet

and exercise, you should get your body composition tested at the beginning of the Healthy You! program and again following the 14-day plan. If you incorporate physical activity into the program, you will most likely not only see a drop on the scale, but in your body fat percentage as well. Many local health clubs provide body composition/body fat testing for a nominal fee. You can also determine your percentage at home by purchasing body fat calipers online for as little as $3.99; most come with simple-to-follow instructions.

Keeping a journal is another great way to track your progress, a habit that also serves as an effective weight loss tool. Journaling or maintaining a food log makes you more aware of what you're eating so that you can stay on track with healthier habits.

CNN recently ran a story about a woman who credits journaling for her 100-plus-pound weight loss. Charmaine, who went from 260 to 130 pounds, claims that recording her progress in writing demanded that she be honest with herself. Tracking her food intake helped her to lose weight and, most importantly, to keep it off.

According to Marisa Moore, registered dietitian and spokeswoman for the Academy of Nutrition and Dietetics, journaling can provide you with a "personal road map to weight loss, healthier eating and behavior change."

Did You Know?
In a study by the Kaiser Permanente Center for Health Research, participants who kept a food diary or journal lost almost twice as much weight as those who didn't.

Simply writing down what you eat can encourage making better choices. It also helps to reduce or eliminate mindless eating. Purchase a notebook or use the journal provided in Appendix IV and track your meals. There are even applications for your smartphone! Or, as discussed previously, make your own online journal public. Sharing your success with others can really motivate you and make you feel accountable.

CHAPTER 13

Get Physical

Although I'm a big proponent of exercise, the Healthy You! program does not require it. Just the thought of physical activity deters some people from attempting a healthy eating program, so I have developed a program that also works without exercise.

Although you can successfully lose weight without exercising on the Healthy You! program, you can accelerate your weight loss by also incorporating a very manageable exercise program. The decision rests with you. Just remember, the Healthy You! program is rooted in more than weight loss; it's about leading an overall healthier life. As you know, physical activity is an important part of creating and maintaining a strong, well-balanced lifestyle. You may feel compelled to first lose some weight before starting an exercise program, but I do encourage you to make time for exercise in the near future.

Did You Know?
According to the Mayo Clinic, exercise (or regular physical activity) can help prevent or manage certain health problems such as stroke, type 2 diabetes, depression, arthritis and certain types of cancer. Exercise also improves your mood, boosts energy and promotes better sleep, not to mention helps to prevent excess weight gain and to maintain weight loss.

One of the craziest stories I've ever heard about someone starting an exercise program was also one of the most inspiring. We featured Sarah Ducloux-Potter in *Women's Running* magazine. Sarah wanted to start exercising, but she thought her husband and daughter would laugh if they saw her out running through the neighborhood. So instead, she started by running around her kitchen table when her family wasn't home. Sarah said, "I'm sure I looked 100 times more ridiculous jogging around our table!"

Sarah didn't tell her family about her exercise program until she could complete an entire hour of running around her kitchen table. Not only did Sarah's family support her, but once she was brave enough to run outside in public, she also found support by joining her local running club. Training with a group has kept her motivated. She says, "Running has changed my life in so many ways. I've become more comfortable in my own skin."

Sarah utilized a unique mode of starting an exercise program, but it clearly worked for her. No matter what exercise you choose or where you decide to do it—in your own house, at a gym or outside in nature—the most important thing is that you start. Finding someone or a group to exercise with like Sarah did can undoubtedly help encourage you to exercise.

After I graduated from college and moved to New York, finding a workout partner really helped me get back on an exercise program. I had gained so much weight after college that I no longer had the motivation. The last thing I wanted to do was to put on shorts and be seen at the gym. But one night while talking to my roommate, I learned that she was also trying desperately to lose weight. After sharing our stories of dieting peaks and valleys, we made a pact to get up early three to four days a week to run together in Central Park. At first, the change seemed impossible. What would have been an easy jog in my younger years, now left me feeling exhausted and completely out of shape. But we took things slowly and stuck to the routine and, after a few weeks, I started noticing that I had more energy at work and could sleep better than I had in months.

More surprisingly, I soon found myself not craving the late night pizza in the office conference room. I started making healthier food choices, and the weight I had gained started to come off. My roommate and I took the next step and decided to sign up for a local 5K race. The excitement of having a concrete goal kept us motivated to continue our morning runs and also helped encourage healthier food choices. I can't remember my final time in the 5K, but I do still remember that feeling as I crossed the finish line. My hard work had not only paid off, but it left me wanting more. I began to see the appeal of prolonged satisfaction—feeling fit and healthy—versus the short-term gain that came with overindulging and making poor food choices.

Did You Know?
Physical activity leads to feelings of self-empowerment. A study published in *Research Quarterly for Exercise and Sport* examined previously sedentary women as they participated in a physical activity program. Those who followed the program for at least six months were more likely to make it a priority to feel good about themselves, while those who did not stick with the program reported more negative self-talk, feelings of insecurity and a fear of failure. In other words, one of the best ways to adopt a "can do" attitude is to simply get moving!

It doesn't matter whether you start an exercise program at the same time you commence Healthy You! or wait until you have completed the program. What counts is that you make exercise a consistent part of your life. Even incorporating a short walking program into your schedule can reap amazing benefits.

PART FOUR

The Real World

CHAPTER 14

Be Realistic

I know that planning and cooking meals takes time, and I also know there often isn't enough time in the day to accomplish our current list of tasks. Adding extra steps like food shopping and meal preparation can be challenging. That said, I would hate if a lack of time prevented you from achieving your goals of healthier eating and weight loss. If you can follow the program to a "T", then by all means do so, and you'll see quick results. However, if you're going to find the meal preparation too challenging, that's okay too; simply make some adjustments.

With a four-year-old, a six-year-old and a full-time job, I am often too exhausted to cook at the end of the day. However, I've found that I can still reap the benefits of the Healthy You! program thanks to some minor tweaks. I typically pick one or two of my favorite dinner recipes and make extra servings so I can serve them two days in a row. I love the rice pasta primavera, and both my husband and I are happy to eat the dish for consecutive meals. The same goes for the herb chicken and several other options. I've also found that some of the lunch recipes make great dinners too. For example, I will prepare a big batch of vegetarian chili and have it for dinner and then again for lunch the following day. Not only does this save time, but it also allows me to spread out the enjoyment of my favorite meals.

If I've had a really rough day, I've even been known to make a Healthy You! breakfast for dinner. I enjoy scrambled eggs or a veggie omelet in the evenings, and preparing these dishes often takes only a fraction of the time it would to make an actual dinner.

Lastly, I suggest finding one or two restaurants near your home or workplace that can make you a Healthy You!-approved meal. I frequent several eateries near my office that will serve grilled fish and steamed vegetables or a large salad with grilled chicken. I've been known to eat lunch out several days in a row without going off the plan; it's all about knowing how to order. For example, one of my favorite restaurants in downtown St. Petersburg, Fla., serves a grilled tilapia with cream sauce, grilled asparagus and buttermilk mashed potatoes—definitely not a Healthy You!-approved combination. But by simply requesting that the fish come without any sauce, the vegetables be steamed without oil or butter and the buttermilk mashed potatoes be replaced with a plain baked potato or even better a small side salad, the meal has been transformed into one that adheres to the program.

I know many diet programs don't allow any substitutions or flexibility, but I believe that your current circumstances should dictate what's best for you. I love sushi, and I've actually made my own sushi twice—both times for special occasions (a sushi making party and a sushi class at our golf and tennis club). Although a recipe for sushi exists in the Healthy You! program, sushi making can be time consuming. If you have the hours to spare, the process can be a lot of fun, but if you're crunched for time, go ahead and order sushi from your favorite restaurant or local market. Although premade sushi may contain a small amount of sugar in the sushi rice, I still allow myself the delicacy. I realize that real life doesn't always allow for "perfect" behavior, and having a premade sushi roll remains a healthy option.

Here are a few real life tips that can make the Healthy You! program more manageable for those severely crunched for time:

- Make extra dinner servings to have for lunch the next day
- Eat breakfast for dinner—making scrambled eggs in the evening is a quick and easy alternative to preparing a full meal
- Have the same lunch two days in a row, or eat a simple lunch for dinner
- Find one or two restaurants near your home or work that can prepare a Healthy You!-approved meal
- Try to follow the program as best you can, but be realistic and take your personal situation into account

CHAPTER 15

Beyond Week Two

I'm sure that people exist who eat a perfectly clean diet all the time, but I'm definitely not one of them. The good news? You don't have to adhere to a 100% clean diet 365 days a year. You can still lead a healthy lifestyle, maintain an ideal weight and even lose pounds if you sometimes indulge in your favorite foods. To avoid feeling deprived, just be sure to indulge in moderation.

Once you've completed the two weeks, continue consuming previously eliminated food moderately, and pay attention to how your body reacts to the reintroduction of some of the eliminated foods. (For example, you may find that you feel fine after adding wheat back into your diet, but that dairy upsets your stomach.) Put thought into your culinary choices. When adding back wheat, choose whole grains. Choose whole wheat bread instead of white. Choose brown rice over white. For meat, choose organic meat whenever possible, and select lean cuts. If you want to enjoy an alcoholic beverage, choose wine over a higher-calorie mixed drink. You may discover that you feel so good after completing the Clean Phase that you want to continue this way of eating, allowing you to healthfully drop additional weight.

Remember that, after week two, you choose how to move forward. However, if you still have 20 or more pounds to lose, I suggest staying on the Clean Phase for at least one more week.

But if you do choose to reintroduce some of the eliminated foods, try incorporating meals from the Healthy You! program alongside your own recipes.

While some people start to feel so good and to drop weight so quickly by the end of week two that they want to continue to eat clean, others, no matter the positive progress, can't fathom another day without one of the eliminated foods. (I understand how they feel!) Again, this is the beauty of the Healthy You! program; the two weeks provide a jump start on your weight loss while simultaneously giving you the tools to change your eating habits for life.

While completely eliminating alcohol or red meat for longer than the Clean Phase might be too extreme, many people who've completed the program choose to give up artificial sweeteners and processed foods and to at least reduce their intake of red meat and alcohol. Two weeks of healthier eating often prove enough to forever change the way you look at what you put into your body.

No matter what you decide as you complete the Clean Phase, listen to your body as you proceed. You may find that you feel better without wheat in your diet, or perhaps dairy makes you feel congested or bloated. By slowly clearing your system of sugar, wheat, dairy, processed foods and other questionable products you will better understand the likelihood of specific foods negatively affecting your body. Although I love bread, pizza and pastries, I've learned that my body doesn't deal well with an overabundance of wheat (moderation is fine, but too much causes stomach discomfort). I found that as long as I only eat wheat at one meal a day (rather than all three), I feel fine.

Should you find yourself slipping back into old, unhealthy eating habits after completing the 14-day Healthy You! program, simply recommence the 14-day plan. Another week on the Elimination Phase plus another on the Clean Phase will get you back on track.

It's often difficult for participants to know how to proceed after finishing the program. Many are fearful of returning to old eating patterns. To help you make good decisions beyond week two, I've developed a list of healthy food options. See the list in Appendix III. It's entirely up to you what you choose to reintroduce. To summarize, I consume wheat, dairy, sugar and alcohol in moderation and only on occasion, and I have tried to drastically reduce or completely eliminate my intake of red meat, artificial sweeteners and highly processed foods. Based on my personal experience, the cleaner your diet, the more weight you'll continue to lose and the healthier you'll feel.

Beyond Week Two Tips:
- Stay on the Clean Phase for additional quick and healthy weight loss
- Reintroduce some of the eliminated foods, but do so in moderation
- Make healthy selections whenever possible
- Continue to eat clean as often as you can
- Continue to eliminate or reduce the foods that had the biggest negative impact on your health and well-being (or made you feel unwell when reintroduced)
- When preparing your own meals, refer to Appendix III for a list of Healthy You!-approved foods

CHAPTER 16

Occasional Indulgences

The Healthy You! program isn't a fad diet. Instead, it provides a new way to permanently alter your way of thinking about food—a philosophy rooted in being kind to your body and fueling it with meals that are healthy and wholesome.

If you're like me, though, you have your favorite indulgences—perhaps pizza, ice cream, cookies or chocolate. It's difficult to imagine a life devoid of these treats. I'm not willing to give up my favorite junk foods forever, and I don't expect you to either. The key to indulging while still losing or maintaining weight is to allow just one indulgence no more than once per week. This once-a-week exception helps me eat a mostly clean diet without feeling deprived. Stick to the Healthy You! program as outlined, but know that after you've completed the 14-day plan, you'll be able to indulge in moderation once again.

There are psychological and physiological benefits to allowing yourself a weekly indulgence. Psychologically speaking, the knowledge of not being able to have something suddenly makes that item even more appealing and often the focus of one's desires. If you've ever told a child not to do something or not to go somewhere, you'll notice that they tend to focus almost solely on what they've been asked not to do. As adults, we have these same tendencies. Tell me I can't have it, and all I can think about is how much I want it!

I've learned that once I ban my favorite junk foods, I crave them even more. Allowing myself my favorite not-so-healthy treats enables me to eat a relatively clean diet for the long-term without ever truly feeling like I'm on a diet.

> **Did You Know?**
> Allowing one indulgence a week can help you stick with your healthy eating plan for the duration of the week.

Every diet I've ever tried and failed has featured a list of forbidden foods such as chocolate, pizza and alcohol. For some reason, even if I didn't particularly crave those certain foods before commencing the diet, I desperately wanted them once I began and this would sabotage my efforts. With Healthy You!, knowing that after the initial two weeks, I can incorporate some of my favorite foods into my schedule has given me the incentive to persevere with the program.

I find it completely unrealistic to tell someone who has eaten pizza, ice cream, chips or chocolate for years that they can never again enjoy that food. The objective of the Healthy You! program is to encourage a cleaner diet and provide you with the tools you need to make better selections in the real world. Good habits coupled with occasional indulgences can be the key to long-term weight loss.

For me, picking one day a week to indulge—a day that never fluctuates regardless of my schedule—gives me the motivation I need to eat clean and healthy the rest of the week. I've found that people who pick Saturday or Sunday as their cheat day tend to be more successful than those who pick weekdays. When you allow yourself to indulge on a weekend day, you feel ready to start fresh on Monday. People who pick a day during the week often find that they want to indulge again during the weekend. My advice: pick one day, and stick to it. If you pick Saturday and then have a party to attend one Friday, don't switch your cheat day. Stick with the program on Friday, and allow yourself to cheat on Saturday. Make healthy choices at the party with the knowledge that you can indulge in your favorite treat the following day.

Allowing yourself to indulge without guilt in your not-so-healthy preferred foods only works if done in moderation. Select one meal or snack during which to incorporate your favorite foods, and keep the rest of the meals that day clean. If you're craving pancakes for breakfast, go ahead and eat them, but then go back to eating a healthy lunch, dinner and snacks. If you want pizza for dinner, that's fine, just make sure you had a healthy breakfast and lunch and that you controlled your portions. Feel like a piece of double chocolate cheesecake for dessert? Go for it! Just make sure your other meals for the day were free of sugar, wheat and dairy and share the dessert if possible.

I want to emphasize that the plan does not condone an all-you-can-eat meal splurge. Even though you may have any food you desire (and I mean anything), you still need to watch your portions. If you want pizza once a week, then have a slice or two, but don't eat the whole pie. If you're craving chocolate cake then have a slice for dessert, but don't eat the whole cake. If you're craving a juicy piece of steak, then go ahead and have a four- or six-ounce filet, but don't order the 32-ounce porterhouse. If you stick to a normal serving size of your favorite food, you can still lose weight and feel great even when fitting in decadent bites of pizza, ice cream, cake, cookies, steak and pasta.

However, you may feel so good with your new clean eating habits, that you don't care to incorporate any unhealthy foods. The choice is yours. For me, allowing myself to indulge once a week (at one meal) sufficiently satisfies my cravings. The great thing about following the Healthy You! program is that I can eat clean most of the time but still indulge in moderation and maintain my goal weight or even continue to lose weight.

Before doing the Healthy You! program, I suffered from

post-indulgence guilt. While living in New York, I walked by a bakery as I was heading to my apartment. In the window display, I saw the largest cupcakes I had ever seen (if they could even be called "cupcakes"). A mere cup couldn't contain these tremendous treats, which were as large as a cereal bowl and required a two-handed grip.

I stopped to admire them for a moment and then kept walking. But I couldn't get those giant cupcakes out of my mind. I quickly reversed and made a beeline for the bakery's front door. Once inside, I selected the biggest of the big—chocolate, of course, topped with a thick, rich swirl of buttercream icing. I probably would have bought two if the clerk hadn't recognized me from my appearances on Martha Stewart's show.

Within minutes of leaving the shop, I devoured my super cupcake. It tasted even better than it looked! As soon as I had finished the last delicious bite, though, I started to feel guilty. Back then, such guilt had the tendency to send me spiraling down into a multi-day, bad food binge. I thought that since I had already gotten my feet wet, so to speak, I may as well dive in. Over the next few days, the cupcake would be followed by servings of chocolate, cookies and maybe even a pint of mint chocolate chip ice cream.

Fortunately, with the help of the Healthy You! program, I've accepted that it's both impossible and unnecessary to eat healthy all the time. I've learned to consider having a piece of cake or a few cookies every so often as a reward for eating a healthy diet the majority of the time. Now I can put my giant cupcake episodes into proper perspective. Instead of slipping into a guilt-ridden junk food fest, I encourage myself to enjoy a little treat now and then, since I find that these treats often motivate me to make my next meal a healthy one.

Whenever I broach this topic during one of my speaking engagements, people approach me afterward to express their empathy and to share their own quirky eating tales. No matter how hard we try, none of us is perfect when it comes to eating healthily all the time. Slipping up now and again shouldn't make us feel defeated. We can indulge in cookies, cake or even a giant cupcake, as long as we're eating a healthy, well-balanced diet most of the time.

This philosophy makes the Healthy You! program sustainable. The initial two weeks provide you with the foundation for clean, healthy eating, and, by allowing yourself to indulge on occasion, you no longer feel like a prisoner to a diet. You can stick to the program far beyond the 14 days while continuing to enjoy your favorite foods.

What happens after the two-week program is up to you. If followed correctly you can lose 10 to 20 pounds or more. If you have 20 plus pounds to still lose, I encourage you to stay on the Clean Phase. Whether you choose to continue eating clean after the two-week period or you choose to reintroduce some of the eliminated foods, I would suggest incorporating a day when you can guiltlessly enjoy a favorite food. This weekly indulgence does not pertain to the initial two weeks but can become an important ingredient in your long-term success.

I realize it's somewhat counterintuitive to promote clean eating and then suggest people splurge on occasion, but as I mentioned earlier, I don't believe anything should be completely restricted. I think it's realistic to assume that most people are going to indulge every now and then anyway. So by freely allowing yourself this option, you remove the guilt that threatens to sabotage your weight loss.

For more than ten years, I've been able to stay within three or four pounds of my goal weight by indulging on occasion (usually on a weekend). Even when I treat myself, my meals still consist of mostly HealthyYou!-approved meals. I've found that I can maintain my goal weight as long as I stick to the relatively clean diet the rest of the time and as long as I indulge at one sitting each week rather than during an entire day of unhealthy eating.

My cheat day may look something like this:

Breakfast
Two-egg omelet with tomato, onion and spinach
Small fresh fruit salad

Lunch
Large salad with grilled chicken or fish

Snack
Vegetables and hummus

Dinner (Indulgence meal)
Flatbread margarita pizza
Tiramisu

As you can see, I ate a HealthyYou! breakfast, lunch and snack. At dinner, I cheated with a flatbread pizza and dessert, but since the rest of the day had been healthy, I should maintain my goal weight despite the splurges. However, had I not yet reached my ideal weight, I would have chosen either the flatbread or the tiramisu (not both).

In summary, you can have your cake and eat it too, just as long as you make smart choices most of the time, and don't eat the entire cake.

Ask Dawna

I work in an environment where my co-workers bring in candy and junk food on a regular basis, and I have a hard time saying no to sweets. How can I lose weight when there is temptation all around me?

I've been in your shoes, and I know how hard it can be to pass up fresh-baked cookies, candy, etc. First, tell your co-workers that you're trying to eat better and ask them if they would like to join you on your healthy eating quest.You never know; your co-workers may also want to lose weight or eat better. They may just need a little push to get started. If this isn't the case, and the junk food keeps coming in, you will need to find a way to say "no thank you." What worked for me was telling myself that, come Saturday, I could have anything I wanted as long as I said "no thank you" at the office. I love carrot cake. It's by far one of my favorite desserts. So if I promised myself that on Saturday I could enjoy a piece of decadent carrot cake, I would somehow find the willpower to turn down the junk food in the office—which is rarely ever as good as my favorite carrot cake, anyway. I know this might sound like a little mind game, but I found that it really worked. Try it; it could work for you too.

CHAPTER 17

Real Life Challenges

Whether you're traveling on business or visiting family for the holidays, stepping away from your normal routine can wreak havoc on weight loss goals. Although it may take some additional planning, once you know what to do, you'll find it easy to stick to a healthy eating plan.

Restaurants, room service and airplane meals, holiday and office parties—some of the biggest complaints I hear revolve around the challenge of eating healthy away from home. The key while traveling is to simply plan ahead.

It's often difficult to find healthy options on the road. Fast food is the norm for long car trips, and airport food isn't always the healthiest. You can, however, set yourself up for success by following a few simple tips:

- Pack your own healthy meal or snacks
- Drink plenty of water
- Don't get on the plane or arrive at a party hungry
- Keep at least two of your three daily meals clean and healthy
- Skip the buffet
- Offer to bring a side dish or dessert to social gatherings
- Have the food you purchase prepared your way

Pack Your Own Healthy Meal or Snacks

Packing your own snacks ensures that you'll have healthy options when hunger strikes. I typically bring along fresh fruit and nuts or, if I have access to a small cooler bag, sliced vegetables and dip. On longer flights, I've even been known to pack a large garden salad and my favorite Healthy You!-approved dressing.

Drink Plenty of Water

If you're embarking on a long car or airplane ride, make sure you drink plenty of water. Especially when flying, it's easy to get dehydrated, and thirst can often be confused for hunger. Drinking plenty of water will help encourage good choices and deter you from overeating. (Not to mention, drinking water is important to your overall health and weight loss.)

Don't Go Hungry

Before getting on a plane or going to a cocktail party, have a healthy snack or meal so you won't feel compelled to overindulge or make poor choices. The worst thing you can do is show up to a party ravenous and find only options like "pigs in a blanket," sliders and breadsticks.

Eat Two Healthy Meals a Day

It used to be that a weeklong vacation would set me back for several weeks. These days, I actually return from most vacations without having gained an ounce. I've found that following a few simple rules allows me to keep my weight in check while still enjoying my vacation.

If you want to maintain your weight while traveling, turn down the hotel mini-bar key and ask that an empty refrigerator be brought to your room. Fill the fridge with water and healthy snacks.

Vacation perks often include fancy dinners and mixed drinks. I certainly take pleasure in eating and drinking while on vacation, but I make sure to keep breakfast and lunch extremely healthy so I can go a little overboard in the evenings.

I've found that if I stay away from the breakfast buffet and instead eat scrambled eggs and fruit or oatmeal in the morning plus a big salad with a lean piece of meat or a grilled piece of fish for lunch, I can still enjoy a fancy dinner and drinks without gaining any weight. However, once I indulge at every meal, I begin to pack on the vacation pounds.

Avoid the Buffet

For many, going to the buffet gives license to overeat. It's often difficult to have restraint in the presence of so many options. The sheer abundance of food plus beautiful displays have the power to pull us in. In fact, a University of Pennsylvania study suggests that a food's presentation and the variety of colors offered may affect the amount of food we eat. In one study, participants given three flavors of yogurt ate 23% more yogurt than if given only one flavor. In another study, 105 adults were presented with 16-ounce bowls of M&Ms to eat while watching a pilot TV show. Some bowls contained 10 different colors of M&Ms; others had only seven. The adults given the 10-color bowls ate more M&Ms than the adults given the seven color options.

The advantages of a buffet—abundance, variety and presentation—also happen to be its downfall. Skip the buffet whenever possible, and order off the menu instead. Most restaurants, even those that promote their buffet, will allow you to order off the menu. I call the buffet the "see food" diet—you see food; therefore, you eat it. If the buffet is your only option, and the restaurant doesn't allow a la carte orders, simply load up on fresh or steamed vegetables, garden salad and lean meats.

Offer to Bring Something

Whether you're going to a party or to your relative's house for dinner, offer to bring a side dish, appetizer or dessert. Contributing a healthy dish like shrimp cocktail, vegetables and dip or fruit salad will provide you with at least one healthy option to keep you on track. When I attend a party, I almost always bring a vegetable platter with hummus and guacamole. The host is usually thrilled that I made an effort to bring something, and the platter is always empty at the end of the night.

Dining Out

One of my favorite movies of all time is "When Harry Met Sally." I love the scene where Sally orders her meal with everything on the side: "I'd like the chef salad, please, with the oil and vinegar on the side and the apple pie a la mode. But I'd like the pie heated, and I don't want the ice cream on top, I want it on the side, and I'd like strawberry instead of vanilla if you have it, if not, then no ice cream, just whipped cream, but only if it's real; if it's out of a can, then nothing."

People may poke fun at Sally's ordering technique, but, in reality, making substitutions and ordering sauces on the side can be one of the best ways to enjoy dining out while still maintaining one's weight. Years ago, restaurants may have balked at special requests, but today it's become the norm. In fact, 80% of restaurants with the average meal priced over $25—and 70% of restaurants with the average meal priced under $25—say patrons customize their meals today more than ever.

Did You Know?
According to the U.S. Department of Agriculture, dining away from home comprises nearly half of all U.S. consumer food expenditures.

Tips for dining out:
- Ask for a plain baked potato instead of fries
- Ask for sauces or dressings on the side
- Ask for all vegetables to be steamed
- Go for oil-based dressings rather than cream-based

- Opt for red sauces and fruit salsas instead of cream- or cheese-based ones
- Order a salad and an appetizer instead of an entreé
- If you order a salad or appetizer, share a meal
- Pass up the bread basket (out of sight, out of mind)
- Leave some food on your plate, or ask for a to-go box at the beginning of the meal
- Choose a healthy appetizer like shrimp cocktail or seared ahi tuna
- Satisfy your sweet tooth by ordering sorbet or berries and cream or by sharing a more decadent dessert with others

Order food described on the menu as:
- Grilled
- Baked
- Poached
- Steamed
- Blackened

Skip food on the menu described using words like:
- Buttery
- Basted
- Creamy
- Au Gratin
- Smothered
- Fried
- Crispy
- Stir-fried
- Sautéed

Remember that being healthy isn't something you do every now and then; it's a lifestyle. But you can indulge occasionally to make it sustainable. Just because you're traveling or on vacation doesn't mean you have to throw your healthy living habits down the drain. Follow a few simple tips so that even living in the "real world" can't sabotage your weight loss.

CHAPTER 18

It's Never Too Late

It's never too late to change your lifestyle. Small changes, no matter your current age or fitness level, can drastically impact your overall health. I first met John "The Penguin" Bingham in 1998. I was the president of a sports nutrition company based in San Diego, and John was one of our best customers who later became a good friend and one of the company's ambassadors.

John was in his forties when he finally decided he could make some real changes to his eating habits and his activity level. A self-proclaimed "overweight couch potato with a smoking and drinking habit," John had no idea that he would one day run more than 40 marathons and inspire scores of others to get off their couches. But John set his mind to losing weight, and his "I can do it" attitude helped him surpass his initial goals. Nearly 20 years later and 100 pounds lighter, he's one of the greatest weight loss success stories I've encountered. He'll tell you it all began with the courage to change, prompted by the crucial decision to believe in himself. John is now in his sixties and has impressively kept the weight off.

Often people in their forties, fifties and sixties assume that it's too late to change their behavior and habits. But in fact, this is the perfect time to make changes. Later in life, we finally realize that we truly control our own destinies. Losing weight might not come as quickly or effortlessly as it did in our twenties, but it can be so much more rewarding.

Mary Kay Andrews, a New York Times best-selling author, was in her mid-fifties when she decided to change her diet and curb her emotional eating habits. Although it proved a constant battle, especially while traveling on book tours, Mary Kay managed to lose 70 pounds by eating fresh fruits, vegetables and lean meats as well as by limiting processed foods and sugar—her trigger foods. In the summer, the season when her book deadlines usually occur, she often finds the scale creeping back up. Focusing on a clean diet and drinking plenty of water has enabled her to get back on track.

When I asked Mary Kay what losing weight means to her, she said, "It's about eating healthy, feeling better and having more energy. I want to feel good about myself while I am enjoying life." Mary Kay is a great example of how it's never too late to change your eating habits and to successfully lose weight. Mary Kay changed her life, and so can you!

No matter how much weight you need to lose, no matter how out of shape you feel and no matter your age, the Healthy You! program can help you make sustainable life changes.

CHAPTER 19

You Can Do It!

The Healthy You! program has not only changed my life for the better, but also the lives of those who I have shared it with. I am extremely passionate about the program, and I am confident that it can—once and for all —help you lose weight and feel better about yourself on all levels. Just 14 days on the Healthy You! program can provide the changes you need to ultimately succeed in your weight loss struggle.

Healthy You! isn't a fad diet, nor is it a program that's only sustainable for a short period of time. Quick-fix diets may seem appealing, but unless you learn to eat better, the weight you lose often returns once you revert to your normal eating patterns. Healthy You! is a way of life that helps you lose weight quickly and easily and, most importantly, provides you with the necessary tools to permanently keep the weight off.

Fourteen days on the program will make you more conscious of your self-sabotaging eating habits so that you can make smarter choices, leading you on a lifelong path to a healthier life.

To get the most out of the Healthy You! program, you must first believe that you can achieve your weight loss goal. Once you trust that it's possible, you will have set the foundation for your success. Take a few minutes right now. Close your eyes, and imagine yourself succeeding. Envision stepping on the scale and seeing your ideal number. Say aloud,"I CAN DO

THIS," and really mean it. You can do it. Even if you have completely given up, as I once had, vow to start fresh right now. Believe, because it will happen this time. With the Healthy You! program, you can finally lose weight and attain the body you've always wanted.

Imagine yourself losing the weight, slipping into a smaller size, becoming stronger and leaner, having more energy and becoming a healthier you. If you believe it, you can do it!

If you have questions or need a little extra motivation, you can visit me at dawnastone.com. The Healthy You! program changed my life; now it's your turn to let it change yours!

You Can Do It!

APPENDIX I

Healthy You! Recipes

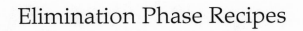

Elimination Phase Recipes

DAY 1 RECIPES

BREAKFAST

Healthy You! Very Berry Smoothie
See page 185 for recipe.

LUNCH

Turkey and Avocado Sandwich

Servings: 1

Ingredients:
2 slices whole wheat or whole grain bread
2 leaves romaine lettuce
2 slices tomato
4 slices cucumber
¼ avocado, mashed
4 thin slices red onion
4 thin slices turkey breast
Spicy mustard (optional)

Directions:
Lay two slices of bread on cutting board and spread half of mashed avocado on one slice. Add turkey, tomato, cucumber, red onion and lettuce. Spread remaining avocado on second piece of bread, and place spread side down on top of sandwich.

DAY 1 RECIPES (Cont.)

DINNER

Grilled Herb Chicken with Steamed Broccoli and Side Salad

Servings: 4

Ingredients:
4 boneless, skinless chicken breasts (organic or hormone-free preferred)
1 tablespoon extra virgin olive oil
1 teaspoon dried oregano
1 teaspoon thyme
1 teaspoon rosemary
½ teaspoon salt
¼ teaspoon garlic, minced
1 head broccoli
4 cups romaine lettuce or European salad blend
8-12 grape tomatoes
2 tablespoons pine nuts
½ cucumber, diced
4 tablespoons Healthy You! dressing of your choice (see pages 187-189 for recipes)

Directions:

Herb Chicken

Preheat grill on medium heat. Lightly oil grates so chicken doesn't stick. Rinse chicken, and place in large resealable plastic bag with olive oil. Seal, and shake. Open bag, and add oregano, thyme, rosemary, salt and garlic. Shake bag to coat chicken. Cook chicken approximately 7-10 minutes on each side, or until thoroughly cooked.

DAY 1 RECIPES (Cont.)

Note: If you don't have access to a grill, place chicken in glass dish, and bake at 350 degrees for approximately 15-20 minutes, or until no trace of pink remains, turning once.

Steamed Broccoli
Rinse broccoli, cut off stalk, and break into bite-size pieces. Bring 1-inch water and salt to boil in saucepan with steamer. Add broccoli, and cover, reduce heat to medium, and cook for 4-6 minutes or until broccoli is bright green and tender.

Note: If you don't have a steamer, steam vegetables directly in water.

Side Salad
Combine salad, tomatoes, pine nuts and cucumbers, and divide onto 4 plates. Drizzle with HealthyYou! dressing.

DAY 2 RECIPES

BREAKFAST

Oatmeal with Fresh Berries and Milk

Servings: 1

Ingredients:
½ cup dry oats (gluten-free, steel-cut oats preferred)
1 ½ cup water
½ cup mixed berries (your choice: blueberries, raspberries, strawberries, etc.)
½ cup sugar-free plain almond milk or ½ cup non-fat milk (optional)

Directions:
Bring water to boil. Add steel-cut oats, and reduce heat to simmer. Cook for 10 – 20 minutes, stirring occasionally. Cover, and remove from heat. Let stand for a few minutes. Top with milk and berries. Enjoy!

Note: If you use rolled oats rather than steel-cut, prepare as directed on package.

LUNCH

Grilled Chicken Caesar Salad

Servings: 1

Ingredients:
2 cups romaine lettuce, torn into bite-size pieces

DAY 2 RECIPES (Cont.)

1 tablespoon Parmesan cheese, shredded
1 small tomato, sliced
1 boneless, skinless chicken breast (organic or hormone-free preferred)
2 tablespoons Healthy You! dressing of your choice (see pages 187-189 for recipes)
Pinch of salt
Pinch of ground black pepper

Directions:
Prepare grill or broiler. Season chicken with salt and pepper. Grill or broil chicken for 15-20 minutes, turning once, or until no trace of pink remains. Cut into strips.

Wash and place salad in bowl, add tomato and cheese and toss with Healthy You! dressing. Add chicken strips.

Note: If you are ordering at a restaurant, substitute balsamic or vinaigrette for Caesar dressing. Also order without croutons.

DAY 2 RECIPES (Cont.)

DINNER

Chicken and Vegetable Stir-Fry over Steamed Brown Rice

Servings: 4

Ingredients:
Extra virgin olive oil spray
4 chicken breasts or chicken cutlets (organic or hormone-free preferred)
1 tablespoon garlic, minced
1 medium yellow onion
1 head broccoli
1 cup snap or snow peas
½ cup baby carrots, julienned
1 bag bean sprouts
1 bag baby spinach, stems removed
2 tablespoons reduced-sodium soy sauce (gluten free/wheat free)*
½ cup water
¼ cup chicken broth (reduced sodium preferred)
¾ cup brown rice
1 pinch salt

Directions:

Stir-Fry
Preheat wok on medium heat, coat with olive oil spray, and combine onion, garlic and soy sauce. Cook 1 minute, then add chicken and chicken broth, and cook for an additional 2-3 minutes. Add carrots, broccoli, snap peas and half of water, and cook for an additional 3-4 minutes. Add bean sprouts, spinach and remaining water, and simmer for an additional 3-5 minutes, or until vegetables are tender and chicken is cooked through.

DAY 2 RECIPES (Cont.)

<u>Rice</u>
Cook rice according to package directions.

Serve stir-fry over rice.

*Most brands of soy sauce contain wheat. You can find wheat-free soy sauce either online or at your local health food store. You may also choose to eliminate the soy sauce from the recipe.

DAY 3 RECIPES

BREAKFAST

Healthy You! Super Green Juice
See page 184 for recipe.

LUNCH

Three Bean Salad

Servings: 4

Ingredients:
1 (15 oz) can northern or cannellini beans, rinsed and drained*
1 (15 oz) garbanzo beans (chick peas), rinsed and drained*
1 (15 oz) can kidney beans, rinsed and drained*
1 large tomato, diced
2 celery stalks, finely chopped
½ red onion, finely chopped
2 tablespoons fresh parsley or cilantro, minced
⅓ cup balsamic vinegar
2 tablespoons extra virgin olive oil
¼ teaspoon salt
¼ teaspoon ground black pepper
1 clove garlic, minced (optional)
1 bag pre-washed mixed greens

Directions:
In small bowl, whisk together balsamic vinegar, extra virgin olive oil, salt, pepper and garlic to create dressing. In large bowl, combine beans, tomato, celery, red onion and parsley. Add dressing to beans, and toss lightly. Refrigerate beans for several hours before serving. Scoop beans over greens, or toss with greens, and enjoy!

DAY 3 RECIPES (Cont.)

Note: The Healthy You! program promotes eating clean and minimally processed food whenever possible. Soaking and cooking dried beans is preferred but often not convenient. I typically use canned beans due to time constraints. When using canned beans, select reduced-sodium and organic options whenever possible.

DAY 3 RECIPES (Cont.)

DINNER

Ginger-Soy Salmon with Steamed Broccoli and Brown Rice

Servings: 4

Ingredients:
4 salmon filets, skin removed
1 teaspoon toasted sesame seeds
½ tablespoon honey (may substitute agavé nectar)
2 tablespoons reduced-sodium soy sauce (gluten free/wheat free)*
1 teaspoon fresh ginger, minced
1 scallion, minced
1 tablespoon rice vinegar
1 head broccoli
Extra virgin olive oil spray
¾ cup brown rice
1 pinch salt

Directions:
Salmon
Combine soy sauce, scallions, honey, ginger and rice vinegar, and stir gently. Place salmon and ½ of marinade in sealable plastic bag. Coat salmon thoroughly, and refrigerate for 10-15 minutes.

Preheat broiler. Cover broiler pan with foil, and spray with olive oil. Transfer salmon to baking pan, and discard marinade. Broil 6-10 minutes, or until cooked through. Transfer to plate, sprinkle with toasted sesame seeds and drizzle with reserved sauce.

DAY 3 RECIPES (Cont.)

Steamed Broccoli

Rinse broccoli, cut off stalk, and break into bite-size pieces. Bring 1 inch water and salt to boil in saucepan with steamer. Add broccoli, and cover, reduce heat to medium, and cook for 4-6 minutes, or until broccoli is bright green and tender.

Rice

Cook rice according to package directions

Most brands of soy sauce contain wheat. You can find wheat-free soy sauce either online or at your local health food store. You may also choose to eliminate the soy sauce from the recipe.

DAY 4 RECIPES

BREAKFAST

Scrambled Eggs and Oatmeal with Almond Milk

Servings: 1

Ingredients:
2 whole eggs
Pinch of salt
¼ teaspoon ground black pepper
Extra virgin olive oil spray
½ cup dry oats (gluten-free, steel-cut oats preferred)
½ cup sugar-free, plain almond milk (optional)

Directions:
Eggs
Whisk together eggs, salt and pepper. Coat non-stick skillet with olive oil spray. Heat skillet on medium heat. Add egg mixture to skillet. Gently scrape eggs around skillet. Cook for 1 to 3 minutes, depending on how well-cooked you like your eggs.

Oatmeal
Bring water to boil. Add steel-cut oats, and reduce heat to simmer. Cook for 10 – 20 minutes, stirring occasionally. Cover, and remove from heat. Let stand for a few minutes. Top with almond milk.

DAY 4 RECIPES (Cont.)

LUNCH

Grilled Salmon and Citrus Salad

Servings: 2

Ingredients:
2 (4 oz) salmon filets, skin removed
3 cups baby spinach, torn stems removed
1 teaspoon honey (optional)
2 tablespoons reduced-sodium soy sauce (gluten free/wheat free)*
½ orange
½ pink grapefruit
¼ cup red onion, thinly sliced
4 tablespoons Healthy You! citrus vinaigrette dressing (see page 188 for recipe)
Extra virgin olive oil spray

Directions:
Combine honey and soy sauce in large sealable plastic bag. Add fish, and shake gently to coat. Place in refrigerator. Preheat broiler. Place fish on broiler pan coated with cooking spray. Broil 13-15 minutes, or until fish flakes easily with fork.

Peel orange and grapefruit. Cut out citrus sections. Combine citrus sections, spinach and red onion evenly on two plates, top with fish, and drizzle with Healthy You! citrus vinaigrette dressing.

Most brands of soy sauce contain wheat. You can find wheat-free soy sauce either online or at your local health food store. You may also choose to eliminate the soy sauce from the recipe.

DAY 4 RECIPES (Cont.)

SNACK

HealthyYou! Strawberry-Banana Smoothie
See page 185 for recipe.

DAY 4 RECIPES (Cont.)

DINNER

Angel Hair Primavera

Serves: 4

Ingredients:
8 oz brown rice pasta (angel hair)
1 cup broccoli, trimmed and cut into bite-size pieces
½ cup mushrooms, sliced
½ cup zucchini, sliced
½ cup yellow squash, sliced
1 clove garlic, minced (optional)
1 large tomato, diced
Salt, to taste
Ground black pepper, to taste
Extra virgin olive oil spray

Directions:
In large pot, bring water to boil, and cook pasta according to package directions. In large saucepan with steamer basket, bring one inch water to boil. Add broccoli, mushrooms, zucchini and yellow squash, and steam until tender. Set aside.

Coat large skillet with extra virgin olive oil spray, and heat on medium. Add tomatoes and garlic, and sauté for 1 minute. Add steamed vegetables, salt and pepper, and cook for an additional minute. Top angel hair with vegetable mixture.

DAY 5 RECIPES

BREAKFAST

HealthyYou! Radiant Red Juice
See page 184 for recipe.

LUNCH

Vegetarian Chili

Servings: 4

Ingredients:
1 tablespoon extra virgin olive oil
1 medium yellow onion, chopped
1 jalapeño pepper, seeded and minced
2 cloves garlic, minced
1 red bell pepper, seeded and chopped
1 tablespoon ground cumin
2 tablespoons chili powder
1 (28 oz) can crushed tomatoes, undrained
1 (15 oz) can tomato sauce
1 cup water (you may add more or less, depending on desired consistency)
1 (15 oz) can black beans, rinsed and drained*
1 (15 oz) can cannellini beans, rinsed and drained*
1 (15 oz) can red kidney beans, rinsed and drained*

Directions:
Place oil in deep pot over medium heat. Add onions and garlic, and sauté for 2-3 minutes, or until onions are translucent. Add jalapeno, bell pepper, cumin, chili powder, tomatoes and tomato sauce. Bring to simmer. Cook 15-20 minutes, stirring

DAY 5 RECIPES (Cont.)

occasionally. Add beans and water. Simmer 25-30 minutes, stirring occasionally.

Note: The Healthy You! program promotes eating clean and minimally processed food whenever possible. Soaking and cooking dried beans is preferred but often not convenient. I typically use canned beans due to time constraints. When using canned beans, select reduced-sodium and organic options whenever possible.

SNACK
Banana and Strawberry Medley

Servings: 1

Ingredients:
1 small banana, sliced
4-6 medium strawberries, sliced

Directions:
In small glass bowl, add alternating layers of bananas and strawberries.

DAY 5 RECIPES (Cont.)

DINNER

Lime-Marinated Flank Steak Over Mixed Greens

Servings: 4

Ingredients:
1 pound flank steak, fat removed
2 limes, squeezed
2 garlic cloves, minced
3 tablespoons balsamic vinegar
1 teaspoon olive oil
¼ teaspoon coarse salt
¼ teaspoon ground black pepper
1 bag pre-washed mixed greens
4 tablespoons Healthy You! white balsamic vinaigrette dressing (see page 187 for recipe)

Directions:
Preheat grill to medium-high heat. In bowl, combine lime juice, garlic, balsamic vinegar, olive oil, salt and pepper. Place steak in sealable plastic bag with marinade, and shake gently to coat. Refrigerate for 10-20 minutes (longer if possible). Remove steaks from marinade, and grill 4-5 minutes on each side. Let cool slightly (5-10 minutes). Slice steak thinly, and place over mixed greens. Drizzle with Healthy You! white balsamic vinaigrette dressing.

Note: You can substitute 4 (4 oz) filet mignon steaks for flank steak.

DAY 6 RECIPES

BREAKFAST
Veggie Omelet and ¼ Melon

Servings: 1

Ingredients:
2 whole eggs
1 egg white
1 small tomato, chopped
2 tablespoons yellow onion, chopped
2 tablespoons green pepper, seeded and chopped
8-10 spinach leaves, washed and stems removed
Pinch of salt
Extra virgin olive oil spray
¼ melon of your choice

Directions:
Whisk eggs in small bowl, and set aside. Coat small non-stick skillet with olive oil spray, and place over medium heat. Add tomato, onion, green pepper and salt, and sauté for 4-5 minutes, or until tender. Transfer vegetables to bowl, and wipe down skillet. Coat skillet with olive oil spray, and place over medium-high heat. Add eggs to skillet, and cook for 2 minutes, lifting edges with spatula to allow uncooked egg mixture to flow to edges and cook. As center of omelet begins to set, add vegetables and spinach to one half of eggs. Use spatula to gently fold one half of eggs over the other. Cook for an additional minute. Serve omelet with sliced melon.

DAY 6 RECIPES (Cont.)

LUNCH

Pasta Salad

Servings: 1

Ingredients:
¾ cup brown rice pasta (shells or fusilli)
1 tomato, chopped
2 scallions, chopped fine
½ head broccoli, cut into small pieces
3 baby carrots, julienned
1 teaspoon Italian seasoning
1-2 tablespoons Healthy You! italian vinaigrette dressing (see page 187 for recipe)

Directions:
Prepare rice pasta as directed on packaging. Wash and cut broccoli and carrots. Place 1 inch water in saucepan, and bring to boil. Place broccoli and carrots in steamer, and cover. Steam on medium-high heat until vegetables are tender. Remove and allow vegetables to cool. Combine cooked rice pasta, tomatoes, scallions, broccoli, carrots and Italian seasoning. Add 1-2 tablespoons Healthy You! italian vinaigrette dressing, toss, cover, and refrigerate for at least one hour.

DAY 6 RECIPES (Cont.)

SNACK

Apple and Natural Peanut Butter

Servings: 1

Ingredients:
1 medium-size apple
1 tablespoon natural peanut butter (natural, no sugar added)

Directions:
Slice apple, and dip or spread peanut butter. Enjoy!

DAY 6 RECIPES (Cont.)

DINNER

Grilled Halibut with Tomato-Mango Salsa, Steamed Asparagus and Brown Rice

Servings: 4

Ingredients:
¾ cup brown rice, uncooked
1 tomato, seeded and diced
½ cup ripe mango, peeled and diced
½ cup red onion, finely chopped
¼ cup fresh cilantro, chopped
2 tablespoons freshly squeezed lime juice
¼ teaspoon salt
Ground black pepper to taste
4 (6 oz) halibut filets
½ tablespoon olive oil
Salt
1 lime
1 lb fresh asparagus

Directions:
Brown Rice
Cook rice according to package directions.

Tomato-Mango Salsa
In medium bowl, combine tomato, mango, red onion, cilantro, lime juice, 1/4 teaspoon salt, and pepper and let stand for 15 to 20 minutes.

DAY 6 RECIPES (Cont.)

Grilled Halibut
Preheat grill or broiler, lightly brush halibut filets with olive oil, and season with salt and pepper. Place fish on grill or in broiler. Cook 5 to 7 minutes per side (make sure fish is opaque at its center).

Asparagus
Clean and cut asparagus. Season lightly with salt, and place in stovetop steamer with boiling water. Steam approximately 4 – 5 minutes, or until tender. (Note: You can also steam in a microwave-safe dish with approximately ¼ cup water. Cover dish and steam for 3 – 5 minutes, or until tender.)

Transfer halibut to plates, and serve with salsa, lime wedge and asparagus.

Note: You can substitute mahi mahi or other white fish for halibut.

DAY 7 RECIPES

BREAKFAST

Spinach, Tomato and Basil Frittata with Fruit Salad

Servings: 4

Ingredients:
6 whole eggs
2 egg whites
6 oz fresh spinach, stems removed
2 tomatoes, thinly sliced and seeded
½ cup onion, finely chopped
½ teaspoon dried basil leaves
½ teaspoon fresh or dried oregano
¼ teaspoon salt
¼ teaspoon ground black pepper
Extra virgin olive oil spray
8 strawberries
8 small chunks cantaloupe
8 small chunks pineapple
8 green or red grapes

Directions:
In large bowl, whisk together eggs, basil, oregano, salt and pepper. Fold in spinach, tomatoes and onion.

Coat non-stick skillet with olive oil spray, and place over medium heat. Pour mixture into skillet. Cook on medium-high. As eggs begin to cook, use spatula to lift edges of eggs, allowing uncooked egg to fill in under cooked parts. Reduce heat, and cook for about 6 minutes, or until the eggs are set. If desired, transfer frittata to preheated broiler for 2 minutes to

DAY 7 RECIPES (Cont.)

lightly brown top. Remove, and let cool for 5 minutes before slicing and serving.

Combine fruit, and serve on plate with frittata.

LUNCH

Cranberry and Quinoa Salad

Servings: 4

Ingredients:
1 cup uncooked quinoa, rinsed
½ cup dried cranberries
2 scallions, finely chopped
¼ cup toasted almonds, sliced
¼ cup fresh cilantro, chopped
1 tablespoon fresh parsley, chopped
2 tablespoons fresh squeezed lemon or lime juice
2 tablespoons extra virgin olive oil
¼ teaspoon ground coriander
¼ teaspoon ground cumin
⅛ teaspoon salt
⅛ teaspoon cracked black pepper

Directions:
Cook quinoa according to package directions, transfer to bowl and refrigerate. Once cool, combine quinoa, cranberries, scallions, almonds, cilantro and parsley in large bowl. In a separate bowl, whisk together lemon (or lime) juice, olive oil, coriander, cumin, salt and pepper. Pour dressing over quinoa, stirring gently to coat.

DAY 7 RECIPES (Cont.)

SNACK

Vegetables and Hummus

Servings: 2

Ingredients:
1 (15 oz) can garbanzo beans (chick peas), rinsed and drained
1 clove garlic, crushed
2 tablespoons tahini sesame seed paste
2 tablespoons freshly squeezed lemon juice
1 tablespoon olive oil
¾ teaspoon salt
2-4 tablespoons water (use more or less, based on desired consistency)
¼ teaspoon paprika (optional)
8 baby carrots
2 celery, halved
½ cucumber, sliced
½ head broccoli, cut in bite-size pieces

Directions:
In food processor, combine garlic, tahini, lemon juice, olive oil and salt. Blend for 30 seconds. Scrape mixture from sides of food processor. Add half of garbanzo beans, and blend for 1 minute. Scrape mixture from sides, and add remaining garbanzo beans. Add water for desired consistency.

Sprinkle with paprika, and serve with fresh vegetables. Cover and refrigerate any leftover hummus.

DAY 7 RECIPES (Cont.)

Note: Feel free to substitute one vegetable for another. For example, sub-stitute ½ a yellow bell pepper for cucumber or ½-head of cauliflower for broccoli. Also, if you are under time constraints and can't make homemade hummus, use a store-bought version.

DAY 7 RECIPES (Cont.)

DINNER

Chicken Soft Tacos

Servings: 4

Ingredients:
1 pound boneless, skinless chicken breast (organic or hormone-free preferred)
2 tablespoons taco seasoning
4 tablespoons freshly squeezed lime juice
8 soft corn tortillas, warmed
¼ cup tomatoes, chopped
1 cup lettuce, shredded
2 tablespoons yellow onions, chopped
1 small avocado, sliced
Hot sauce (optional)

Directions:
Preheat oven to 350 degrees. Combine chicken and taco seasoning in sealable plastic bag. Shake to coat chicken. Pour lime juice in rectangular glass baking dish. Add chicken, and cook 15-20 minutes, or until chicken is cooked thoroughly. Cut chicken into small pieces. Fill warm tortillas with chicken, tomatoes, lettuce, onions and avocado. Add hot sauce. Fold, and enjoy.

Clean Phase Recipes

DAY 8 RECIPES

BREAKFAST

HealthyYou! Super Green Juice
See page 184 for recipe.

LUNCH

Grilled Chicken and Chickpea Garden Salad

Servings: 1

Ingredients:
1 boneless, skinless chicken breast (organic or hormone-free preferred)
Pinch of salt
Pinch of ground black pepper
2 cups romaine lettuce, torn into bite-size pieces
1 small tomato, sliced
4 thin slices, red onion (optional)
4 thin slices, green bell pepper
¼ cucumber, sliced
½ cup chickpeas, drained
2 tablespoons HealthyYou! dressing of your choice (see pages 187-189 for recipes)

Directions:
Prepare grill, or preheat broiler. Season chicken with salt and pepper. Grill or broil chicken for 15-20 minutes, turning once or until no trace of pink remains. Cut chicken into strips.

Wash and place salad and remaining ingredients in bowl, and toss with HealthyYou!-approved dressing. Top with chicken.

DAY 8 RECIPES (Cont.)

SNACK

Tortilla Chips and Fresh Salsa

Servings: 4

Ingredients:
8 corn tortillas (wheat-free brand)
3 tomatoes, chopped
½ cup onion, finely chopped
1 jalapeño, minced (optional for spicy salsa)
¼ cup fresh cilantro, minced
2 tablespoons freshly squeezed lime juice
Salt, to taste

Directions:

Tortilla Chips
Slice each tortilla into 4-6 triangular sections. Preheat oven to 350 degrees. Place tortillas on baking sheet and cook until tortillas are just beginning to brown. Remove, sprinkle with salt and let cool.

Salsa
Combine all ingredients in bowl, and refrigerate for a few hours before serving.

Note: Salsa tastes best if left in the refrigerator overnight.

DAY 8 RECIPES (Cont.)

DINNER

Crab Cakes and Green Beans

Servings: 4

Ingredients:
1 pound cooked crabmeat, lump
2 egg whites
2 shallots, finely chopped
¼ cup green or red bell pepper, finely chopped
¼ cup sugar-free, plain almond milk
2 tablespoons spicy mustard, prepared (not dry)
2 tablespoons parsley, finely chopped
1 teaspoon Chesapeake Bay seasoning
1 teaspoon ground white pepper
Extra virgin olive oil spray
2 tablespoons oat flour for dusting work surface
1 pound fresh green beans, cut into 2-inch segments
Salt

Directions:
Crab Cakes
Combine in large bowl crabmeat, egg whites, shallots, bell pepper, almond milk, mustard, parsley, Chesapeake Bay seasoning and pepper. Mix together gently. Form into 8 small cakes. Place flour on cutting board, and lightly coat each cake on both sides.

Spray large non-stick skillet with olive oil spray. Cook crab cakes on medium heat until golden, turning once (approximately 4-6 minutes on each side).

DAY 8 RECIPES (Cont.)

Green Beans

Clean, and cut off ends of green beans. Place in stovetop steamer with boiling water. Steam approximately 4-5 minutes, or until tender. Sprinkle with salt.

DAY 9 RECIPES

BREAKFAST

Healthy You! Pineapple-Avocado Smoothie
See page 186 for recipe.

LUNCH

Vegetable Soup* and Salad

Servings: 4

Ingredients:
64 oz reduced-sodium vegetable broth (organic preferred)
2 leeks, sliced
10 oz fresh green beans, pre-cut if desired
10 oz fresh carrots, pre-cut if desired
1 teaspoon dried thyme
Ground black pepper, to taste
1 (14 oz) can fire-roasted diced tomatoes
3 small to medium zucchini squash, sliced
10 oz fresh cauliflower, pre-cut if desired
4 cups romaine lettuce or European salad blend
8-12 grape tomatoes
1 teaspoon sunflower seeds
4 tablespoons Healthy You! dressing of your choice (see pages 187-189 for recipes)

Directions:
Vegetable Soup
Add leeks and green beans to broth, and bring to boil for 10 minutes. Add carrots, thyme, pepper and fire-roasted tomatoes.

DAY 9 RECIPES (Cont.)

Bring back to boil, then simmer for 30 minutes. Add 3 small to medium zucchini squash plus cauliflower, and continue to simmer for additional 30 minutes, or until vegetables are tender.

Note: This is the recipe of my sister, Michele, a very busy single mom. Although homemade vegetable soup tastes delicious, it can demand a lot of preparation time. For convenience, this soup is made with pre-cut and bagged vegetables, canned tomatoes and boxed or canned vegetable broth, which you can purchase at your local grocery store. However, as an alternative, you can cut your own vegetables and make your own vegetable stock.

Side Salad
Combine lettuce, tomatoes and sunflower seeds. Divide onto 4 small plates, and add one tablespoon Healthy You! dressing per salad.

SNACK

Celery and Natural Peanut Butter

Servings: 1

Ingredients:
2 stalks celery
1 tablespoon natural peanut butter (natural, no sugar added)

Directions:
Cut stalks in half, spread peanut butter on stalks. Enjoy!

DAY 9 RECIPES (Cont.)

DINNER

Black Bean Tostadas

Servings: 4

Ingredients:
8 corn tortillas
2 (15 oz) cans black beans, rinsed and drained
¼ cup hot sauce
2 tablespoons water
½ cup tomatoes, diced
½ avocado, diced
1 tablespoon onions, minced
1 tablespoon jalapenos, minced (optional)
⅛ teaspoon salt
2 teaspoons freshly squeezed lime juice

Directions:
For salsa, combine tomatoes, avocado, onions, jalapenos, salt and lime juice in a small bowl, and set aside.

Combine hot sauce, water and black beans in blender or food processor, and blend until smooth. Heat bean mixture in saucepan on low-medium heat or in microwave-safe bowl for 1-2 minutes.

Preheat oven to 350 degrees. Place tortillas on baking sheet or directly on oven rack, and bake for 3-5 minutes on each side, or until tortilla is crispy and starts to brown.

Top tortillas with black bean mixture, lettuce and salsa.

DAY 10 RECIPES

BREAKFAST

HealthyYou! Strawberry-Banana Smoothie
See page 185 for recipe.

LUNCH

Lentil Salad*

Servings: 4

Ingredients:
1 cup lentils (green or brown)
2 cups water
1 bay leaf
Coarse salt, to taste
Ground black pepper, to taste
1 clove garlic, minced
2 medium carrots, peeled and diced
½ medium red onion, finely chopped
2 tablespoons extra virgin olive oil
3 tablespoons red wine vinegar
¼ cup fresh parsley, finely chopped
1 cup arugula
1 cup endive
Extra virgin olive oil spray

Directions:
Wash lentils thoroughly. Combine lentils, water and bay leaf in saucepan. Bring to boil over medium-high heat. Once boiling, reduce to gentle simmer. Cook uncovered for 20-30 minutes, or until lentils are tender. If needed, add more water. Strain

DAY 10 RECIPES (Cont.)

lentils, remove bay leaf, and return to saucepan or bowl, and add salt and pepper. Spray large skillet with olive oil spray. Heat on medium, and add garlic, carrots and red onion. Cook about 4-5 minutes, until carrots are tender and onions are translucent. Add mixture to lentils. Add extra virgin olive oil and red wine vinegar, and stir to coat lentils. Add parsley, and serve over arugula and endive mixture.

*Can be served warm or cold.

Tip for the workplace: Make lentils the night before. Refrigerate lentils overnight, and microwave at the office the next day. After microwaving lentils, serve over arugula and endive mixture.

DAY 10 RECIPES (Cont.)

DINNER

Agavé Rosemary Chicken and Wild Rice

Servings: 4

Ingredients:
¾ cup wild rice, uncooked
4 boneless, skinless chicken breasts, cut in strips (organic or hormone-free preferred)
2 cloves garlic, minced
1 tablespoon dried rosemary or 2 tablespoons fresh rosemary, finely chopped
1 tablespoon agavé nectar or honey
1 tablespoon Dijon mustard
Salt, to taste
Ground black pepper, to taste
Extra virgin olive oil spray

Directions:
Wild Rice
Cook rice according to package directions, and set aside.

Agavé Rosemary Chicken
Spray large, non-stick skillet with olive oil spray, and heat over medium-high heat. Season chicken with salt and pepper, and add chicken, garlic and rosemary to skillet. Cook 4-6 minutes on each side, or until chicken is cooked through.

Add cooked rice, agavé nectar (or honey) and Dijon mustard. Cook additional 2-3 minutes, stirring occasionally to coat chicken and rice thoroughly.

DAY 11 RECIPES

BREAKFAST
Veggie Scramble and Oatmeal

Servings: 1

Ingredients:
2 whole eggs
½ cup spinach, stems removed
½ cup tomatoes, diced
¼ cup onion, diced
Salt, to taste
Ground black pepper, to taste
Extra virgin olive oil spray
½ cup dry oats (gluten free, steel cut preferred)

Directions:
Eggs
Whisk eggs, salt and pepper, and set aside. Coat non-stick skillet with olive oil spray, and heat on medium. Add spinach, tomatoes and onion, and sauté until tender. Pour egg mixture over vegetables. Gently scrape eggs around skillet. Cook for 1 to 3 minutes, depending on how well-cooked you like your eggs.

Oatmeal
Bring water to boil. Add steel-cut oats, and reduce heat to simmer. Cook for 10 – 20 minutes, stirring occasionally. Cover, and remove from heat. Let stand for a few minutes. Enjoy!

DAY 11 RECIPES (Cont.)

LUNCH

Walnut and Pear Salad

Servings: 2

Ingredients:
4 cups baby spinach, stems removed
½ fennel bulb, thinly sliced (optional)
1 pear, sliced
¼ cup walnuts, roughly chopped
¼ cup red onion, thinly sliced
¼ cup mushrooms, sliced
2 tablespoons raisins
4 tablespoons Healthy You! walnut vinaigrette dressing (see page 188 for recipe)

Directions:
In bowl, combine spinach, fennel, pear, walnuts, red onion, mushrooms and raisins. Toss with Healthy You! walnut vinaigrette dressing.

SNACK

Healthy You! Magic Mango Smoothie
See page 186 for recipe.

DAY 11 RECIPES (Cont.)

DINNER

Fish Tacos with Mango-Avocado Salsa

Servings: 4

Ingredients:
1 pound halibut or mahi mahi filets
8 corn tortillas, warmed
1 cup cabbage, shredded
1 tablespoon freshly squeezed lime juice
1 avocado, sliced
1 mango, chopped
2 tablespoons red onion, diced
2 tablespoons fresh cilantro, chopped
Ground black pepper, to taste
Salt, to taste
Extra virgin olive oil spray

Directions:
Combine lime juice, avocado, mango, red onion and cilantro in medium bowl, and let sit. Coat large non-stick skillet with olive oil spray. Season fish with salt and pepper, and place on skillet. Cooking time will depend on thickness of fish, but should be about 3 minutes on each side, or until fish is barely translucent. Place fish and cabbage in warm tortillas, add salsa, fold, and enjoy!

DAY 12 RECIPES

BREAKFAST

Healthy You! Radiant Red Juice
See page 184 for recipe.

LUNCH

Greek Salad with Grilled Chicken

Servings: 2

Ingredients:
2 boneless, skinless chicken breasts (organic or hormone-free preferred)
4 cups romaine lettuce, torn into bite-size pieces
1 tomato, sliced
8-10 Kalamata olives
½ cucumber, seeded and chopped
½ green bell pepper, seeded and chopped
¼ cup red onion, finely chopped
4 tablespoons HealthyYou! Greek dressing (see page 189 for recipe)
Ground black pepper, to taste
Salt, to taste

Directions:
Prepare grill, or preheat broiler. Season chicken with salt and pepper. Grill or broil chicken for 15-20 minutes, turning once, or until no trace of pink remains. Cut chicken into strips.

Combine lettuce, tomato, olives, cucumber, green bell pepper and red onion in large bowl. Toss with Healthy You! Greek dressing. Top with chicken, and serve.

DAY 12 RECIPES (Cont.)

DINNER

California Roll (Sushi) with Edamame

Servings: 4 rolls

Ingredients:
1 cup sushi or short grain rice (brown rice optional)
2 ½ cups water
2 tablespoons rice vinegar
½ tablespoon salt
4 crab sticks
1 medium avocado, peeled, pitted and sliced into 1/8-inch slices
3 tablespoons freshly squeezed lemon juice
4 sheets unseasoned nori
1 cucumber, seeds removed and julienned
Toasted sesame seeds
Pickled ginger for garnish
Wasabi for garnish
Reduced-sodium soy sauce for dipping (gluten free/wheat free)*
2 cups edamame (soy beans in pods, fresh or frozen)

Directions:
Sushi Rice
Place rice in bowl, and rinse with water. Repeat until water is clear. Place rice and water into medium saucepan. Bring to boil, uncovered. Turn heat to low, cover, and simmer for additional 15 minutes, or until water has been absorbed. Remove from heat, and let stand for 10 minutes. Combine rice vinegar and salt, and heat in microwave for 30 seconds. Fold vinegar mixture into rice, making sure to coat each grain. Cool at room temperature before making sushi.

DAY 12 RECIPES (Cont.)

Sushi

Gently toss avocado in lemon juice to prevent browning. Cover bamboo sushi mat with plastic wrap. Have small bowl of water available. Wet fingers with water, and spread approximately ½ cup rice evenly onto nori. Sprinkle rice with sesame seeds. Turn nori rice side down, and place cucumber, avocado and crab sticks in center of sheet. Roll nori evenly, holding crab, cucumber and avocado in place while rolling. Cover with damp cloth or towel, and continue with other rolls. Cut each roll into 6-8 pieces, and serve with soy sauce, ginger and wasabi.

Edamame

Steam or microwave according to package.

Most brands of soy sauce contain wheat. You can find wheat-free soy sauce either online or at your local health food store. You may also choose to eliminate the soy sauce from the recipe.

Note: If you have a busy schedule and don't have time to make your own sushi, purchase some at your local market or sushi restaurant. However, be aware that many establishments use sugar in their sushi rice. Should you want to eat 100% clean for the 14 days, you may want to use the sugar-free recipe above. Restaurant sushi can still be part of a healthy diet.

DAY 13 RECIPES

BREAKFAST

Veggie Omelet and Fresh Fruit Cup

Servings: 1

Ingredients:
2 whole eggs
1 egg white
1 small tomato, chopped
2 tablespoons yellow onion, chopped
2 tablespoons green pepper, seeded and chopped
8-10 spinach leaves, stems removed
Salt, to taste
Extra virgin olive oil spray
2 strawberries, sliced
4 small pineapple chunks
4 small cantaloupe chunks (or other melon)

Directions:
Whisk eggs in small bowl, and set aside. Coat small non-stick skillet with olive oil spray, and place over medium heat. Add tomato, onion, salt and green pepper, and sauté for 4-5 minutes, or until tender. Transfer vegetables to bowl, and wipe down skillet. Coat skillet with olive oil spray, and place over medium-high heat. Add eggs to skillet, and cook for 2 minutes, lifting edges with spatula to allow uncooked egg mixture to flow to edges and cook. As center of omelet begins to set, add vegetables and spinach to one half of eggs. Use spatula to gently fold one half of eggs over the other. Cook for additional minute.

Combine fruit on plate with omelet, and serve.

DAY 13 RECIPES (Cont.)

LUNCH

Wild Rice and Spinach Soup

Servings: 4

Ingredients:
3 cups water
1 cup wild rice, uncooked
1 teaspoon olive oil
1 cup onion, chopped
2 garlic cloves, crushed
2 carrots, coarsely chopped
1 celery stalk, chopped
3 tablespoons tomato paste
1 teaspoon dried basil
1 teaspoon dried oregano
3 (16 oz) cans reduced-sodium chicken broth (organic, if possible)
1 (14 oz) can diced tomatoes, un-drained
3 cups spinach, torn (stems removed)
¼ teaspoon salt
¼ teaspoon ground black pepper

Directions:
Wild Rice
Cook rice according to package directions.

Soup
In Dutch oven, heat oil over medium heat. Add onions and garlic, and sauté for 1 minute, or until onions are translucent. Add 3 cups water, carrots, celery, tomato paste, basil, oregano, chicken broth and diced tomato. Bring to boil, reduce

DAY 13 RECIPES (Cont.)

heat, and simmer 20-30 minutes. Add cooked rice, spinach, salt and pepper, and simmer for additional 3 minutes.

SNACK

Vegetables and Hummus

Servings: 2

Ingredients:
1 (15 oz) can garbanzo beans (chick peas), rinsed and drained
1 clove garlic, crushed
2 tablespoons tahini sesame seed paste
2 tablespoons freshly squeezed lemon juice
1 tablespoons olive oil
¾ teaspoon salt
2-4 tablespoons water (use more or less, based on desired consistency)
¼ teaspoon paprika (optional)
8 baby carrots
2 celery, halved
½ cucumber, sliced
½ head broccoli, cut in bite-size pieces

Directions:
In food processor, combine garlic, tahini, lemon juice, olive oil and salt. Blend for 30 seconds. Scrape mixture from sides of food processor. Add half of garbanzo beans, and blend for 1 minute. Scrape mixture from sides, and add remaining garbanzo beans. Add water for desired consistency.

DAY 13 RECIPES (Cont.)

Sprinkle with paprika, and serve with fresh vegetables. Cover, and refrigerate any leftover hummus.

Note: Feel free to substitute one vegetable for another. For example, substitute a yellow bell pepper for cucumber or ½ head of cauliflower for broccoli. Also, if you are under time constraints and can't make homemade hummus, use a store-bought version.

DAY 13 RECIPES (Cont.)

DINNER

Mushroom Risotto

Servings: 4

Ingredients:
1 cup Arborio rice or other risotto rice
1 cup mushrooms of your choice (crimini, shitake, etc.)
4 cups chicken or vegetable broth (organic and reduced sodium preferred)
1 tablespoon olive oil
2 cloves garlic
¾ cup shallots, chopped
¼ teaspoon salt

Directions:
In saucepan, warm broth on low heat. Heat olive oil in medium-large saucepan over medium-high heat. Add mushrooms, shallots and garlic, and cook until shallots are translucent (approximately 2 to 3 minutes). Add rice and salt to the mushroom mixture, and stir to coat. Stir ½ cup hot broth into rice mixture, and cook on medium-low heat, stirring constantly. When broth is almost completely absorbed, add another ½ cup hot broth, and continue to stir. Repeat until all broth has been absorbed in ½ cup increments. Expect 30 to 45 minutes of total cooking time.

DAY 14 RECIPES

BREAKFAST

HealthyYou! Super Green Juice
See page 184 for recipes.

LUNCH

Crab, Mango and Avocado Stack

Servings: 4

Ingredients:

1½ - 2 cups crab meat (jumbo, lump preferred)
1 cup tomatoes, diced
1 cup cucumber, diced
1 cup mango, diced
1 cup avocado, diced
2 cups spring mix, washed
1 food ring or empty can
4-6 tablespoons Healthy You! citrus vinaigrette dressing (see page 188 for recipe)

Directions:

Crab Stack

To create stack, you will need a food ring for a mold (if you do not have food ring, you can use a tin can with both top and bottom removed as a mold). Place mold on serving plate. Begin layering ingredients into mold, ¼ of each crab, mango, avocado, cucumber and tomato. Press down while slowly removing mold. Repeat with remaining ingredients to create four molds—each on separate plate. Place ½ cup spring mix on each plate, and drizzle Healthy You! citrus vinaigrette dressing over spring mix and crab stack.

DAY 14 RECIPES (Cont.)

DINNER

Fish in Parchment with Pineapple-Mango Chutney, Basmati Rice and Asparagus

Servings: 4

Ingredients:
4 large pieces parchment paper
4 (4-6 oz) halibut filets
1 tablespoon water
Salt, to taste
Ground black pepper, to taste
1 teaspoon extra virgin olive oil
1 lemon, thinly sliced
2 teaspoons dried or fresh thyme
1 cup basmati rice
1 bunch asparagus spears
½ cup pineapple, chopped
½ cup mango, chopped
½ cup cucumber, finely chopped
¼ cup onion, minced
½ jalapeno, minced
4-6 fresh mint leaves
¼ cup seasoned rice wine vinegar

Directions:
Halibut
Preheat oven to 400 degrees. Fold each piece of parchment in half, and cut each into heart shape. Coat or spray each side of parchment paper with olive oil. Place halibut filet in middle of one side of parchment. Add water. Sprinkle with salt and

DAY 14 RECIPES (Cont.)

pepper. Drizzle with olive oil, and top with 2 slices of lemon and thyme. Repeat for 3 remaining filets.

Fold paper heart in half, and tightly fold over edges to form seal. Transfer to baking sheet, and bake for 15 minutes. Remove from oven, and let stand for 5 minutes. Serve in parchment.

Pineapple-Mango Chutney
Combine pineapple, mango, cucumber, onion, jalapeno, mint and rice wine vinegar in a refrigerator safe covered dish. Refrigerate for 20 – 30 minutes (longer for a stronger flavor). Serve over fish.

Basmati Rice
Cook rice according to package directions.

Steamed Asparagus
Trim ends off asparagus. In large saucepan with steamer, bring one inch water to boil. Add asparagus, and steam for 5-10 minutes, or until asparagus is tender. Remove, and sprinkle with salt.

Healthy You!
Juices, Smoothies and Dressings

HEALTHY YOU! JUICES

HEALTHY YOU! SUPER GREEN JUICE

Servings: 1

Ingredients:
4 large kale leaves
1 small green apple
1 stalk celery
½ cucumber
½ lemon

Directions:
In a juicer, juice all ingredients and serve in tall glass. If you enjoy your juice really cold, pour over ice.

HEALTHY YOU! RADIANT RED JUICE

Servings: 1

Ingredients:
1 cup mixed berries
1 small green apple
1 stalk celery
½ cucumber
½ lemon
1 cup spinach

Directions:
In a juicer, juice all ingredients, and serve in tall glass. If you enjoy your juice really cold, pour over ice.

HEALTHY YOU! SMOOTHIES

HEALTHY YOU! VERY BERRY SMOOTHIE

Servings: 1

Ingredients:
2 strawberries
¼ cup blueberries or raspberries
½ banana
½ cup almond milk
4 ice cubes (optional)

Directions:
Place all ingredients in blender, and blend until smooth.

HEALTHY YOU! STRAWBERRY-BANANA SMOOTHIE

Servings: 1

Ingredients:
4-5 strawberries, fresh or frozen
½ banana
½ cup almond milk
2 tablespoons freshly squeezed orange juice
4 ice cubes

Directions:
Place all ingredients in blender, and blend until smooth.

HEALTHY YOU! SMOOTHIES (Cont.)

HEALTHY YOU! PINEAPPLE-AVOCADO SMOOTHIE

Servings: 1

Ingredients:
½ avocado
½ banana
¼ cup pineapple
½ cup water
4 ice cubes

Directions:
Place all ingredients in blender, and blend until smooth.

HEALTHY YOU! MAGIC MANGO SMOOTHIE

Servings: 1

Ingredients:
½ mango, peeled, diced and frozen
½ banana
½ cup almond milk
2 tablespoons freshly squeezed orange juice
4 ice cubes

Directions:
Place all ingredients in blender, and blend until smooth.

HEALTHY YOU! DRESSINGS

WHITE BALSAMIC VINAIGRETTE

Makes approximately ½ cup

Ingredients:
6 tablespoons white balsamic vinegar
2 tablespoons extra virgin olive oil
1 tablespoon Dijon mustard
¼ teaspoon salt
⅛ teaspoon ground black pepper

Directions:
Combine white balsamic vinegar, extra virgin olive oil, Dijon mustard, salt and ground black pepper. Whisk, and refrigerate.

ITALIAN VINAIGRETTE

Makes approximately ½ cup

Ingredients:
3 tablespoons extra virgin olive oil
3 tablespoons red wine vinegar
1 tablespoon freshly squeezed orange juice
1 ½ teaspoon Dijon mustard
1 teaspoon garlic, minced
Salt, to taste

Directions:
Combine extra virgin olive oil, red wine vinegar, freshly squeezed orange juice, Dijon mustard, garlic and salt. Whisk, and refrigerate.

HEALTHY YOU! DRESSINGS (Cont.)

CITRUS VINAIGRETTE

Makes approximately ½ cup

Ingredients:
2 tablespoons freshly squeezed lemon juice
2 tablespoons freshly squeezed orange juice
2 tablespoons extra virgin olive oil
3 tablespoons red wine vinegar
1 tablespoon Dijon mustard
¼ teaspoon salt
Ground black pepper, to taste

Directions:
Combine lemon juice, orange juice, extra virgin olive oil, red wine vinegar, Dijon mustard, salt and ground black pepper. Whisk, and refrigerate.

WALNUT VINAIGRETTE

Makes approximately ½ cup

Ingredients:
2 tablespoons walnut oil
4 tablespoons white wine vinegar
2 tablespoons lemon juice
¼ teaspoon salt

Directions:
Combine walnut oil, white wine vinegar, lemon juice and salt. Whisk, and refrigerate.

HEALTHY YOU! DRESSINGS (Cont.)

GREEK DRESSING

Makes approximately ½ cup

Ingredients:
4 tablespoons extra virgin olive oil
4 tablespoons red wine vinegar
4 teaspoon dried oregano
Salt, to taste
Ground black pepper, to taste

Directions:
Combine olive oil, red wine vinegar, dried oregano, salt and ground black pepper. Whisk, and refrigerate.

Accelerate Your Results

We all know the saying "slow and steady wins the race." However, I've learned from experience that losing weight too slow can cause you to lose motivation. You may give up just days into a weight loss program because you're not seeing immediate or quick results. In reality, we want results, and we want them fast! The Healthy You! program will give you quick results that will keep you motivated to stay on the program.

If, like me, you have an "all or nothing" personality, you may choose the accelerated program. Although the regular program will still lead to fast results, the accelerated program will likely have you dropping a few extra pounds during week one. If seeing even more immediate weight loss will help keep you motivated, then the accelerated program may be more suitable for you.

The accelerated program consists of only one minor (but important) difference from the regular two-week program, yet it also requires a bit more willpower and self-control. The program isn't as easy as the regular two-week program but you will see results much quicker.

As you've learned by now, the two phases that comprise the regular Healthy You! program are: Elimination and Clean. On the accelerated program, simply skip the Elimination Phase, and begin with the Clean Phase. Therefore, you will eat clean for the entire two-week period.

If you choose the accelerated program, follow the meal plan beginning on page 194 during week one. You will notice that it varies only slightly from the regular week 1 meal plan and that all recipes can be found in the regular 14-day program. Follow the regular Clean Phase meal plan for the second week of the accelerated program.

Whether you choose to follow the regular two-week program or to jump straight into the two-week accelerated program, you will quickly drop those unwanted pounds.

Accelerated Meal Plan

	Day 1	Day 2	Day 3	Day 4	Day 5	Day 6	Day 7
Breakfast	Healthy You! Very Berry Smoothie	Oatmeal with Fresh Berries & Almond Milk	Healthy You! Super Green Juice	Scrambled Eggs & Oatmeal with Almond Milk	Healthy You! Radiant Red Juice	Vegetable Omelet & 1/4 Melon	Spinach, Tomato & Basil Frittata with Fruit Salad
Lunch	Walnut & Pear Salad	Grilled Chicken Salad	Three Bean Salad	Grilled Salmon & Citrus Salad	Vegetarian Chili	Pasta Salad	Cranberry & Quinoa Salad
Snack (optional)	Small Handful Green or Red Grapes	Medium-Size Apple and 10 Raw Almonds	Medium-Size Apple or Pear	Healthy You! Strawberry-Banana Smoothie	Banana & Strawberry Medley	Medium-Size Apple & 1 TBSP Peanut Butter	Vegetables & Hummus
Dinner	Grilled Herb Chicken with Steamed Broccoli and Side Salad	Chicken & Vegetable Stir-Fry Over Steamed Brown Rice	Ginger-Soy Salmon with Steamed Broccoli and Brown Rice	Angel Hair Primavera	California Roll (Sushi) with Edamame	Grilled Halibut with Tomato-Mango Salsa, Asparagus & Brown Rice	Chicken Soft Tacos
Eliminated items:	Sugar, Wheat, Dairy, Highly Processed Foods, Diet Soda and Artificial Sweeteners, Red Meat and Alcohol	Sugar, Wheat, Dairy, Highly Processed Foods, Diet Soda and Artificial Sweeteners, Red Meat and Alcohol	Sugar, Wheat, Dairy, Highly Processed Foods, Diet Soda and Artificial Sweeteners, Red Meat and Alcohol	Sugar, Wheat, Dairy, Highly Processed Foods, Diet Soda and Artificial Sweeteners, Red Meat and Alcohol	Sugar, Wheat, Dairy, Highly Processed Foods, Diet Soda and Artificial Sweeteners, Red Meat and Alcohol	Sugar, Wheat, Dairy, Highly Processed Foods, Diet Soda and Artificial Sweeteners, Red Meat and Alcohol	Sugar, Wheat, Dairy, Highly Processed Foods, Diet Soda and Artificial Sweeteners, Red Meat and Alcohol

Detailed accelerated meal plan starts on page 194 and recipes can be found in Appendix I

DAY 1

OPTIONAL ACCELERATED MEAL PLAN

BREAKFAST

Healthy You! Very Berry Smoothie

LUNCH

Walnut and Pear Salad

SNACK

Small Handful Green or Red Grapes

DINNER

Grilled Herb Chicken with Steamed Broccoli and Side Salad

DAY 2

OPTIONAL ACCELERATED MEAL PLAN

BREAKFAST

Oatmeal with Fresh Berries and Almond Milk

LUNCH

Grilled Chicken Salad

SNACK

Medium-Size Apple and 10 Raw Almonds

DINNER

Chicken and Vegetable Stir-Fry over Steamed Brown Rice

DAY 3

OPTIONAL ACCELERATED MEAL PLAN

BREAKFAST

Healthy You! Super Green Juice

LUNCH

Three Bean Salad

SNACK

Medium-Size Apple or Pear

DINNER

Ginger-Soy Salmon with Steamed Broccoli and Brown Rice

DAY 4

OPTIONAL ACCELERATED MEAL PLAN

BREAKFAST
Scrambled Eggs and Oatmeal with Almond Milk

LUNCH
Grilled Salmon and Citrus Salad

SNACK
Healthy You! Strawberry-Banana Smoothie

DINNER
Angel Hair Primavera

DAY 5

OPTIONAL ACCELERATED MEAL PLAN

BREAKFAST

Healthy You! Radiant Red Juice

LUNCH

Vegetarian Chili

SNACK

Banana and Strawberry Medley

DINNER

California Roll (Sushi) with Edamame

DAY 6

OPTIONAL ACCELERATED MEAL PLAN

BREAKFAST

Veggie Omelet and ¼ Melon

LUNCH

Pasta Salad

SNACK

Medium-Size Apple and 1 Tablespoon Peanut Butter (Natural, No Sugar Added)

DINNER

Grilled Halibut with Fresh Tomato-Mango Salsa, Steamed Asparagus and Brown Rice

DAY 7

OPTIONAL ACCELERATED MEAL PLAN

BREAKFAST

Spinach, Tomato and Basil Frittata with Fresh Fruit Salad

LUNCH

Cranberry and Quinoa Salad

SNACK

Vegetables and Hummus

DINNER

Chicken Soft Tacos

Healthy You! Approved Foods

Although you don't have to worry about what to eat during the 14-day Healthy You! program, thanks to the detailed daily meal plan, I encourage you to continue to eat clean following the two-week program. In order to help you make good selections, I have included a list of Healthy You! clean foods. Note that only the most common or most easily found options have been listed below. Use this list as a way to experiment with new foods while still maintaining a clean and healthy diet.

Vegetables
There are a plethora of vegetables available, so think outside the box when stocking up. Some of the most common and easily found include:

Alfalfa Sprouts
Artichoke
Arugula
Asparagus
Bean Sprouts
Broccoli
Brussels Sprouts
Cabbage
Carrots

Cauliflower
Celery
Chicory
Chives
Collard Greens
Corn
Cucumber
Eggplant
Endive
Fennel
Garlic
Ginger
Green Beans
Green Pepper
Jicama
Kale
Leek
Lemon Grass
Lettuce
Mushrooms
Mustard Greens
Okra
Onion
Parsley
Parsnip
Peas
Potato
Pumpkin
Radicchio
Radish
Red Pepper
Rhubarb
Romaine Lettuce
Scallions
Shallots

Soy Beans
Spaghetti Squash
Spinach
Spring Greens
Squash
Sugar Snap Peas
Sweet Potato
Turnip
Water Chestnut
Watercress
Yam
Yellow Pepper

Fruits
Find below a list of the most readily available fruits:

Apple
Apricot
Avocado
Banana
Blackberry
Blueberry
Cantaloupe
Cherry
Clementine
Coconut
Cranberry
Cumquat
Fig
Grapefruit
Grapes
Guava
Honeydew Melon
Kiwi Fruit
Lemon

Lime
Mango
Olive
Orange
Papaya
Passion Fruit
Pear
Persimmon
Pineapple
Plum
Pomegranate
Prickly Pear
Prune
Raisin
Raspberry
Star Fruit
Strawberry
Tangerine
Tomato
Watermelon

Note: Fruit can be highly caloric and, although a natural sugar, most still contain a high sugar content. Keep your fruit consumption to one serving at a time. For example, eat a small piece of fruit or a cup of berries rather than a large bowl of fruit salad. Note that a large piece of fruit often constitutes two servings.

Whole Grains
Find below a list of healthy wheat-free grains:

Amaranth
Brown Rice
Millet
Oats (Gluten Free, Steel Cut)
Quinoa

Rice Pasta
Teff
White Rice
Wild Rice

Legumes
Find below a list of healthy legumes:

Black Beans
Black Eyed Peas
Cannellini Beans
Edamame
Garbanzo Beans (Chick Peas)
Great Northern Beans
Kidney Beans
Lentils
Pinto Beans
Red Beans
Split Peas

Nuts and Seeds
Find below a list of healthy and common nuts and seeds:

Almonds
Cashews
Pecans
Pumpkin Seeds
Pine Nuts
Sesame Seeds
Sunflower Seeds
Walnuts

Meats and/or Proteins
Find below a list of HealthyYou!-approved meats/proteins:

Chicken
Eggs
Fish
Turkey

Oils
Find below a list of oils that are Healthy You! approved:

Extra Virgin Olive Oil (used in moderation and not for frying)
Grapeseed Oil
Sesame Oil
Walnut Oil

HEALTHY YOU! JOURNAL

As mentioned earlier, keeping a journal is a great way to track your progress; the practice can serve as an extremely effective weight loss tool. Journaling or recording in a food log keeps you aware of what you're putting in your body, helps reduce mindless eating and allows you to consistently maintain healthier habits.

Use the following journal pages as a simple way to track your progress during the 14-day Healthy You! program.

ELIMINATION PHASE, DAY 1

Date:_____

Morning Weight:_____ *(Optional)*

	Time	Meal Description	Other Notes
Breakfast			
Lunch			
Snack			
Dinner			

ELIMINATION PHASE, DAY 2

Date:_____

Morning Weight:_____*(Optional)*

	Time	Meal Description	Other Notes
Breakfast			
Lunch			
Snack			
Dinner			

ELIMINATION PHASE, DAY 3

Date:_____

Morning Weight:_____ *(Optional)*

	Time	Meal Description	Other Notes
Breakfast			
Lunch			
Snack			
Dinner			

ELIMINATION PHASE, DAY 4

Date:_____

Morning Weight:_____*(Optional)*

	Time	Meal Description	Other Notes
Breakfast			
Lunch			
Snack			
Dinner			

ELIMINATION PHASE, DAY 5

Date:_____

Morning Weight:_____*(Optional)*

	Time	Meal Description	Other Notes
Breakfast			
Lunch			
Snack			
Dinner			

ELIMINATION PHASE, DAY 6

Date:_____

Morning Weight:_____ *(Optional)*

	Time	Meal Description	Other Notes
Breakfast			
Lunch			
Snack			
Dinner			

ELIMINATION PHASE, DAY 7

Date:_____

Morning Weight:_____*(Optional)*

	Time	Meal Description	Other Notes
Breakfast			
Lunch			
Snack			
Dinner			

CLEAN PHASE, DAY 8

Date:_____

Morning Weight:_____*(Optional)*

	Time	Meal Description	Other Notes
Breakfast			
Lunch			
Snack			
Dinner			

CLEAN PHASE, DAY 9

Date:_____

Morning Weight:_____ *(Optional)*

	Time	Meal Description	Other Notes
Breakfast			
Lunch			
Snack			
Dinner			

CLEAN PHASE, DAY 10

Date:_____

Morning Weight:_____ *(Optional)*

	Time	Meal Description	Other Notes
Breakfast			
Lunch			
Snack			
Dinner			

CLEAN PHASE, DAY 11

Date:_____

Morning Weight:_____ *(Optional)*

	Time	Meal Description	Other Notes
Breakfast			
Lunch			
Snack			
Dinner			

CLEAN PHASE, DAY 12

Date:_____

Morning Weight:_____*(Optional)*

	Time	Meal Description	Other Notes
Breakfast			
Lunch			
Snack			
Dinner			

CLEAN PHASE, DAY 13

Date:_____

Morning Weight:_____ *(Optional)*

	Time	Meal Description	Other Notes
Breakfast			
Lunch			
Snack			
Dinner			

CLEAN PHASE, DAY 14

Date:_____

Morning Weight:_____*(Optional)*

	Time	Meal Description	Other Notes
Breakfast			
Lunch			
Snack			
Dinner			